Nursing diagnosis of the alcoholic person

Nursing diagnosis of the alcoholic person

NADA J. ESTES, R.N., M.S.

Associate Professor, Psychosocial Nursing Department,
Alcohol and Drug Abuse Nursing Program,
University of Washington, Seattle, Washington

KATHLEEN SMITH-DiJULIO, R.N., M.A.

Assistant Professor, Psychosocial Nursing Department,
Alcohol and Drug Abuse Nursing Program,
University of Washington, Seattle, Washington

M. EDITH HEINEMANN, R.N., M.A.

Professor, Psychosocial Nursing Department;
Director, Alcohol and Drug Abuse Nursing Program,
University of Washington, Seattle, Washington

illustrated

The C. V. Mosby Company

ST. LOUIS · TORONTO · LONDON   1980

Printed in the United States of America

The C. V. Mosby Company
11830 Westline Industrial Drive, St. Louis, Missouri 63141

Library of Congress Cataloging in Publication Data

Estes, Nada J   1930-
  Nursing diagnosis of the alcoholic person.

  Includes bibliographical references and index.
    1. Alcoholism—Diagnosis.   2.   Psychiatric nursing.
I.   Smith-DiJulio, Kathleen, 1949-   joint author.
II. Heinemann, M. Edith, 1920-   joint author. III.
Title. [DNLM: 1.   Alcoholism—Diagnosis—Nursing texts.
WY160 E79n]
RC565.E83   616.86′1′075   80-11057
ISBN 0-8016-1558-5

TS/M/M 9 8 7 6 5 4 3 2 1   01/D/054

To **Duane, Annette, Tonya, Don, Carey,** and **Marlene**
for their support when we needed it during
the writing of this book

Preface

Increasingly, in our stressed modern society, people are using mood-altering substances for multitudinous reasons, especially for the relief of anxiety. Alcohol, because of its easy availability, legality, low cost, and general social acceptance, has become the most commonly chosen drug.

Nurses in all spheres of practice frequently encounter persons who use alcohol in harmful ways as well as those whose lives are seriously affected by alcoholic relatives and friends. Approximately 7% of the adult population have problems with alcohol; as a result, people with alcohol problems are often represented in hospitals, clinics, and nursing homes. These people manifest varying degrees of physiologic and psychosocial sequelae resulting from their involvement with alcohol.

It is essential that every nurse possess the knowledge and skills necessary to provide safe and effective care for persons affected by alcoholism. Schools of nursing have a responsibility to provide opportunities for such learning. We realize that the breadth and depth of study may vary from person to person and may be influenced by such factors as interests and levels of or opportunities for study. However, as educators of nurses we believe that all nurses need fundamental knowledge enabling them to prevent and intervene in the development of alcoholism. To do this, they must perform a comprehensive nursing appraisal that provides the basis for diagnosis and for selection and implementation of appropriate management strategies. *Nursing Diagnosis of the Alcoholic Person* is written to facilitate this process. Little, if any, information has been assembled that concentrates primarily on *nursing* appraisal of alcoholic persons and their nonalcoholic family members.

This book is intended to provide the nurse with adequate theoretical background to perform comprehensive and accurate appraisal of alcohol problems in all persons seeking health care. Content about prevention and treatment options, less detailed in nature, is also presented, so that nurses will have background information on which to base the selection of management strategies. Chapter 1 presents a nursing model and then applies it to alcoholism. Conceptual views of alcoholism and the various professionals rendering care to those affected are also discussed in the initial chapter. Chapter 2 provides criteria for defining and diagnosing alcoholism and an overview of theories of causation. The various physiologic and psychosocial aspects of alcoholism are the focus of Chapter 3. The unique features of alcohol problems in special population groups, including racial and ethnic groups, adolescents, multidrug abusers, women, the elderly, and nurses, are addressed in Chapters 4 and 5. Appraisal by interview, including tools, guides, and interview phases, is presented in Chapters 6 and 7, while Chapter 8 covers appraisal by means of physical examination. Chapter 9 presents appraisal data on two alcoholic clients who exhibit contrasting features. The intent of this chapter is to demonstrate how the nurse makes use of appraisal data, derived from the interview and physical examination, to determine nursing diagnoses and management strategies. Chapter 10 deals with intervention in alcohol problems, emphasizing treatment options. Chapter 11 contains tools for appraisal of nonalcoholic family members as well as information about the indirect effects of alcoholism on spouses and children.

We have presented some definitions of alcoholism in Chapter 2, yet there is still no one definition that the entire research and treatment community agrees upon. One purpose of this book is to write about the person suffering deleterious consequences of excessive alcohol consumption whether that consumption pattern is called abuse, alcoholism, or something different. Thus at various times throughout the book we have interchanged the terms abuse and alcoholism. Both indicate use of alcohol to the point where it affects a person's ability to function.

We are well aware that both men and women develop alcoholism and that both men and women are nurses, and some attempt has been made to delete pronouns to avoid bias. However, this has not always been possible or feasible. For expedience, clarity, and readability the alcoholic person is often referred to in the third person, masculine gender, and the nurse in the third person, feminine gender. Individuals with alcoholism are referred to as persons or clients, which in turn emphasizes their humanity and the personal efforts they make to obtain help and achieve health.

We are grateful to Ruth Sivertsen, Program Assistant to the Alcohol and Drug Abuse Nursing Program, University of Washington School of Nursing. Her meticulous typing of the manuscript and her words of encouragement during the arduous process of writing and rewriting it were especially appreciated. The writing of this book was supported in part by Grant No. 67-1024 from the National Institute of Alcohol Abuse and Alcoholism. In addition, we would like to acknowledge the contributions of Nancy Willig, Family Nurse Practitioner, and Dr. James Smith, Director, Schick's Shadel Hospital, Seattle, to the development of Chapter 8. Also, the provision of clinical data and careful delineation of subsequent nursing actions by Jo Anne Cunningham, R.N., M.N., greatly enriched Chapter 9.

Nada J. Estes
Kathleen Smith-DiJulio
M. Edith Heinemann

Contents

CHAPTER 1

Issues affecting the diagnosis of alcoholism

Alcohol is the most abused drug and alcoholism is one of the most serious health problems in the United States. The alcoholic person not only suffers from generalized demoralization and unhappiness but also from serious physical maladies like cirrhosis, gastritis, and brain damage. Alcoholism can shorten the life span of those afflicted by as many as ten to twelve years. People whose lives intertwine with the alcoholic person, including family members, close friends, and work associates, often are adversely affected by alcoholism as well. They repeatedly suffer intense psychologic reactions such as extreme embarrassment, fear, and resentment as a result of close association with a person who is frequently inebriated and hung over.

In the numerous settings where nurses work, they have frequent contact with people who experience alcohol-related problems. Yet, nurses have been reluctant to care for such persons partly because of a general lack of knowledge of alcoholism and because of limited expertise in treating alcoholic persons. Nursing care largely has been provided unsystematically and intuitively. At the same time the chronicity of alcoholism and the labeling of the alcoholic person as difficult to care for have contributed to the nurse's lack of interest. Alcoholism has received low priority in the health care system, and afflicted persons have tended not to seek help and acknowledge their problem in its early stages. Consequently, attempts at treatment have met with minimal success, and many nurses have preferred to work with people who are perceived as having a more hopeful prognosis.

At the same time alcoholism is now recognized by many as a highly treatable entity. Recent advances in its identification and treatment portend hope rather than pessimism regarding the prognosis of those afflicted by this major killer. It is timely and of utmost importance for nurses to become prepared to work effectively with persons who experience alcohol-related problems. Nurses can better meet the challenge of providing quality care to such people by increasing their understanding of alcoholism and its manifestations and by developing expertise in diagnosing alcoholism in its various guises.

In this chapter we present a framework for nursing diagnosis of the alcoholic person, describe conceptual views of alcoholism, and discuss aspects of provision of care to alcoholic persons. In subsequent chapters we expound on the knowledge base and clinical skills necessary to acquire, from the alcoholic person and family, accurate appraisal data, the substantive core from which diagnoses and management strategies are formulated.

NURSING DIAGNOSIS AND MANAGEMENT

Nursing's primary purpose is to assist individuals and their families to achieve their highest possible health status so that they may effectively meet the expectations of their daily lives. To achieve this purpose with persons afflicted by alcoholism, it is necessary first for the nurse to appraise accurately the ways in which alcoholism affects a person's daily life. The formulation of nursing diagnoses and the selection of management strategies follow the accumulation of appraisal data.

The data that any health care practitioner finds useful for understanding a person's problem with alcoholism are similar and include appraisal of high-risk areas on which diagnosis and management are focused. High-risk areas are those aspects of life most likely to be adversely affected by alcoholism. When an alcoholic person is actively drinking excessive amounts of alcohol, high-risk areas include the following:

Physical health

Increased susceptibility to infection
Altered nutritional status
Interference with sleep activity
Interference with sexual activity
Impairment of vital organs
Diminished energy
Increased risk of accident and injury
Substantial reduction in life span
Insufficient exercise

Psychosocial well-being

Low self-concept
Feelings of alienation, guilt, depression, anger
Increased risk of suicide
Increased consumption of other drugs that interact with alcohol
Interferences with interpersonal relationships, including family,
    friends, co-workers
Lack of creative diversion such as hobbies, recreational activities
Thwarted personal growth, learning, and maturity
Delayed development of potential
Lack of philosophical or spiritual pursuits

Economic well-being

Possible loss of job or demotion
Indebtedness

Legal entanglements

Increased incidence of arrest for driving while intoxicated (DWI) or for assaults,
    including child abuse, spouse battering, and tavern fights
Increased likelihood of divorce, and difficulties surrounding custody of children

Factors associated with the diagnosis of alcoholism

Social stigma with regard to alcoholism
Lack of acceptance of the diagnosis by all involved

When drinking diminishes or ceases, as during recovery, risk factors change and primarily center around maintenance and adjustment to modified drinking patterns, including abstinence. Alcoholism is a chronic disease, and the tendency to relapse is especially pronounced during the first year of sobriety. Even when a person is highly motivated to change drinking patterns, the massive alterations required to achieve this goal are often overwhelming. The risk of relapse remains for individuals recovering from alcoholism who live in a society that condones and encourages drinking and that frequently exposes them to opportunities to drink.

Although similar high-risk areas are appraised by various professional disciplines, each discipline makes use of the data obtained somewhat differently. The practical use that nurses make of appraisal data is in determining how best to assist alcoholic persons to improve their health by mobilizing their resources to meet the requirements of daily life more adequately. This involves selecting and implementing management strategies directed toward decreasing the degree of risk to which the person is exposed. This purpose, although not rigid and absolute, constitutes nursing's independent practice.

The theoretic aspects of nursing's *independent* practice are explained in detail elsewhere.[3] A condensation of this theory is presented here in that the content is useful in guiding the nurse to acquire pertinent appraisal data and to determine appropriate management strategies. The theory explicates a model of nursing based on the assumption that *the major purpose of nursing is to enable persons to meet the activities and demands of daily living with their available resources, both internal and external*. To clarify this model, we will define terms and give examples from our experience with alcoholic persons.

Activities of daily living (ADL) are regularly or frequently occurring events in the alcoholic person's pattern of daily living, that is, eating, sleeping, eliminating, shopping, socializing. The activities are important to both the alcoholic person and to those close to him. For example, the alcoholic man's daily trip to the liquor store to purchase alcohol interferes with his family's financial solvency and hence with their ability to purchase necessities such as food and clothing.

Demands of daily living (DDL) are expectations that the alcoholic person and others have that affect choices or feelings about the activities of daily living.[9] The alcoholic man just cited provides an example of the way the demands of daily living operate and how the activities and demands of daily living overlap. As the man makes his daily trip to the liquor store, he expects his wife to berate him for spending the family's money on alcohol, for breaking his promise to her to cut down his drinking, and for failing to accept treatment for his drinking problem. His own expectations are similar to those of his wife. He expects to be able to exert control over his drinking but finds himself failing again and again and succumbing to the desire to drink. Over time his repeated failures lead to a lowering of the expectations he has of himself, causing him to feel guilty, worthless, hopeless, and helpless and thereby increasing his expectation that alcohol will make him feel better.

Internal resources (IR) are the functional capabilities the person is able to mobilize to manage daily living. Internal resources can include physical and emotional well-being, knowledge, skill, desire, and courage.[9]

External resources (ER) are forces and environmental features outside the person, such as housing, neighborhood, interpersonal support systems, professional services, transportation, and finances, that maintain the individual in a preferred or required life-style.[9]

As alcoholism worsens, both internal and external resources diminish. The alcoholic person's ability to solve problems, an internal resource, becomes obscured by defenses, such as denial and projection. Family members and friends, external resources, are likely to become alienated as a result of the alcoholic person's preoccupation with drinking and thus are less available.

These four components of the model, when used as a basis for gathering appraisal data, enable nurses to make clinical judgments leading to diagnosis and management strategies. In addition, the nurse needs to take the alcoholic person's life-style into account in *balancing* the activities and demands of daily living against his internal and external resources. Assisting a client to achieve this type of balance is the essence of nursing. Fig. 1 is a schematic representation of this balance.

The base of the figure represents a person. It can also represent a system, such as a family or community. At any one point the activities and demands of daily living should be in balance with the internal and external resources. This state of balance is achieved by persons experiencing optimum health

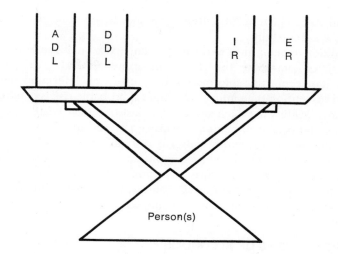

Fig. 1. Nursing model. (Modified from Carnevali, D. L., and Patrick, M.: Nursing management for the elderly, Philadelphia, 1979, J. B. Lippincott Co.)

and by those who have adjusted to adverse alterations in health status. Imbalances occur when activities and demands cannot be managed because of deficits in the internal or external resources or when the resources are insufficiently challenged. The degree of imbalances depends on the severity of the deficit as well as the extent to which another component compensates for the deficit. An example is the alcoholic person with a strong desire to stop drinking but who cannot because of insufficient personal resources. Nurses appraise the client's insufficiencies and determine how to assist him to implement additional resources or to modify existing ones to attain sobriety. When sobriety is achieved, the likelihood of regaining a balance between patterns of daily living and available resources is increased.

This model attempts to clarify nursing's independent practice. Historically, the nursing practice most evident to the general public, and indeed to many nurses, has been its dependent practice, that is, the carrying out of physician's orders. The following example illustrates how the nurse fulfills both independent and dependent practice areas.

An alcoholic person is diagnosed as having peripheral neuropathy. The physician's primary focus is on the nature and extent of the lesion and on its amelioration by thiamine (vitamin B_1). Responsibility for administering thiamine is delegated to the nurse and represents nursing's dependent practice area. The nurse, within her independent area of clinical practice, diagnoses deficits in the client's personal resources, specifically loss of sensation in hands and feet, which in turn alters his ability to meet the requirements of daily living successfully.

In addition to being alert to the degree and extent of loss of sensation, the nurse gathers data about the client's environment and usual patterns of everyday life. From this information the nurse can determine the client's increased susceptibility to injury. The highest probable risk is of injury to the person's extremities in which sensation is lost (physical health) and to self-esteem (psychosocial well-being). The nurse's prescription is directed toward assisting the person to modify patterns of daily living until his functional abilities are strengthened. For example, modifications are indicated in regard to the placing of furniture according to the needs of a person with diminished sensation, paying special attention to safety measures while cooking, smoking, and bathing as well as implementing measures to enhance self-esteem.

CONCEPTUAL VIEWS OF ALCOHOLISM

In addition to understanding the nursing role, the nurse's concept of alcoholism is a factor of considerable importance in the outcome of her interaction with the alcoholic person. Alcoholism, unlike many other conditions, can be looked at from a number of perspectives. Some prevalent conceptual views, namely that it is a moral problem, a disease, or a behavioral aberration, are presented in the following discussion.

Alcoholism, a moral issue

In the early 1800s the Temperance Society was formed in the United States because many persons were concerned about the excessive drinking among the general population. The society was dedicated to the promotion of temperate drinking. When its efforts failed to control the heavy drinking, the emphasis changed to attempts to control the alcohol itself. Thus abstinence became the focus. As a result, conflict arose between manufacturers, distributors, and consumers of alcohol, "the wets," and those who did not use alcohol in any way, "the drys."

As the battle raged, the alcoholics, whose plight had started it all, were forgotten. The evils of alcohol, so ardently preached, were transferred to them; they too were judged evil. And, since very very few of them were able to stop drinking, they were deemed hopeless, and most people simply wrote them off. Only a few doctors, here and there, persisted in trying to help them, with all too little success. Their affliction was considered a disgrace. Worse, it was considered to be their own fault—a self-inflicted condition. Many people believed that alcoholics were simply pleasure-mad, seeking their own pleasure at everyone else's expense. Others believed they were congenital weaklings, somehow subhuman with no backbone, no will power, and no character. They were also considered moral delinquents, people of no basic value at all. Thus alcoholism came to be regarded as strictly a moral problem, and alcoholics as people of no worth. It is not surprising that no constructive action could take place in such an atmosphere. This was the origin of stigma, that smothering blanket which so effectively prevented alcoholics or their families from recognizing, admitting, or seeking help for their illness. [10, p. 6]

Some people today still adhere to this belief and assume that the alcohol abuser is a "willful sinner" who freely chooses to drink. [4] Under this model treatment consists of punishing the sinner, often by placing him in jail and castigating him socially. The alcoholic person treated in this manner can be expected to experience overwhelming feelings of guilt and, in an effort to escape social rejection, is likely to deny his alcoholism. As isolation from friends and family increases, his drinking continues to its most devastating chronic state, often ending in premature death.

The decline of this mode of thought coincided with an increased understanding of the nature of alcoholism. Studies began to provide evidence that contradicted the postulates of the moral concept. It was found, for instance, that not all heavy drinking leads to alcoholism and that some persons seem to have a genetic predisposition to the development of alcoholism. [6] Societal influences and racial differences in reactions to alcohol were identified as possible factors relating to the incidence of alcoholism. [5, 13] Alcoholism became known as a disease entity, and a medical concept emerged.

Alcoholism, a disease

The medical model characteristically defines the origin of disease as arising from within the person and outside volitional control. It assigns major responsibility for provision of treatment to society and health professionals. Under the model, treatment is most appropriately given in health agencies, such as clinics or hospitals, and alcoholic drinking is seen as a symptom of physiologic disturbance. Complete abstinence, removal of the etiologic agent, is seen as the most acceptable means to recovery.

The first description of symptom progression of alcoholism was published in the early 1960s. [7] Since then, many authorities have accepted belief in the disease concept. Alcoholism has been defined as a disease by both the American Medical Association and the American Nurses' Association. This concept has positively influenced early detection and has done much to remove stigma. Without the overwhelming feeling of guilt, prevalent when alcoholism was viewed as a moral problem, alcoholic persons are more able to present themselves for treatment. Treatment facilities have proliferated, and support for research has increased. The increase in research has resulted in new insights along with possibilities of improving services to alcoholic people.

At the same time, shortcomings of the disease concept are recognized.

Critics deplore the tendency to erroneously describe alcoholism as a unitary entity, since current knowledge indicates that it appears to stand for a set of related yet differing disorders. Furthermore, sociocultural factors, which likely influence the development of alcoholism in certain groups of people, are deemphasized. Another important issue inherent in the disease concept is that of shifting the responsibility for treatment away from the affected person. Attempting to relieve the alcoholic person of major responsibilities for treatment is unrealistic in that ultimate responsibility for bringing about changes in the course of alcoholism rests with the affected individual. Another argument against the disease concept is that it has been a self-fulfilling prophecy for some. Such persons have neglected to seek early treatment, claiming that since alcoholism is a disease it is impossible for them to change it, and they readily accept the dictum of "once an alcoholic, always an alcoholic."[1, 14]

Alcoholism, a learned behavior

In contrast with the moral and disease beliefs is the learning model of alcoholism, the focus of considerable current research. From this viewpoint, alcoholism is considered to be acquired and maintained in part by known mechanisms of learning, especially behavioral reinforcement.[11, 12] Learning to use alcohol can occur in numerous ways, including the process of emulation, as children model parental drinking behavior and as adolescents drink along with their peer group. In these instances young people are taught verbally and by example that alcohol is a substance to be used in certain ways to achieve specific desired effects. Group pressure to drink and social recognition and acceptance of drinking in the United States, where alcohol is readily available and frequently used, all influence the manner in which a person learns to drink.

People also learn to use alcohol as a result of experiencing its tension-reducing effects. The example of drinking after a difficult day at the office is a familiar one. The pleasant effects of drinking provide an immediate reinforcement for more drinking so that the pattern of alcohol consumption in response to tension becomes repetitive and overlearned. Whether or not a person learns to depend on alcohol can be viewed as contingent on whether he receives any positive reinforcement from drinking.[2, 4] Alcoholics are identified as persons who initially obtained greater tension release from the use of alcohol than other people and who continue to use it in greater than normal quantities as a learned or conditioned response.

Chronically ill alcoholic individuals experiencing the withdrawal syndrome learn that alcohol temporarily halts the withdrawal process, bringing both relief and further reinforcement of drinking. Drinking is the immediate learned response to the discomfort of withdrawal but is inadequate. In fact, the need for the next drink only becomes more compelling because the entire process is further reinforced. A vicious circle develops that both provokes and perpetuates drinking.

Proponents of the learning model believe that changes to reduce drinking can be achieved and can lead to full recovery from alcoholism. Holding this view as an accepted premise influences the selection of management strategies. When a decrease in drinking behavior is an accepted goal for recovery, treatment focuses on assisting the person to develop new ways of coping with tension rather than relying on excessive alcohol intake to achieve relaxation.

It is only in recent years that the doctrine of complete abstinence, as a necessary premise for the rehabilitation of all alcoholic persons, has come under question. The subject of controlled drinking is a controversial one for those working with alcoholic persons and, of course, for alcoholic persons themselves. In the scientific community numerous questions related to this subject are being raised. Early research findings do not provide conclusive evidence that controlled drinking is a long-term, therapeutically effective goal for all persons. Indeed, proponents of controlled drinking have never suggested that all alcoholic persons are candidates for this treatment. Selection of persons who might benefit is an extremely careful process. Young people are included, since they have not been drinking excessively for many years, they can still remember other ways to consume alcohol, and they are likely not to remain abstinent for the rest of their lives. Also included are persons with strong social support systems, family, friends, and jobs, and those for whom abstinence-oriented treatment approaches have repeatedly failed.

In addition to the moral, disease, and behavioral concepts, there are other models that attempt to explain the emergence of alcoholism. These include psychosocial, cultural, and genetic models, which are discussed in Chapter 2.

It is important for the nurse appraising the alcoholic person to be aware of differing conceptual views and of her own stance with regard to them. At the same time, the nurse needs an awareness of how the alcoholic client and his family view alcoholism. It may be evident that certain views are more common with one alcoholic person than with another. For example, some alcoholic persons have a familial history of alcoholism, whereas others do not. In another instance, a spouse who believes that her alcoholic husband's drinking is a moral problem may think that his recovery depends primarily on his regular involvement in church-related activities. The nurse needs to tailor management strategies to coincide with the client's and family's belief system and life-style, thus increasing the likelihood of his following a management plan.

PROVISION OF CARE TO ALCOHOLIC PERSONS

In addition to the diversity of conceptual views of alcoholism, there is another dimension that affects the appraisal process. Two major groups provide care to alcoholic persons: those who themselves have recovered from alcoholism and those who have never been afflicted. The former, possessing a personal experience of alcoholism and having obtained varying degrees of formal education, constitute an important treatment force. Without advanced education in psychosocial and physiologic areas, the recovered alcoholic care providers primarily have their own experience with alcoholism to guide them in the appraisal, diagnosis, and management process; therefore their emphasis is largely on alcoholism. As a result, their ability to focus on other factors common to alcoholic people, such as marital conflict and psychologic disorders, may be limited.

In addition to the group of recovered alcoholic care providers, nurses, physicians, and other health professionals have become prepared to use their knowledge and skills with alcoholic people. As a rule, these people have not had a personal experience with alcoholism but are interested in working with afflicted persons as a result of their understanding of alcoholism as a major health problem. Applying findings from clinical practice and research, they are beginning to develop strategies toward prevention and are increasingly successful in using effective interventive and rehabilitative procedures.

Whether or not one group or the other is better suited to provide services to alcoholic persons has not been resolved. Since alcoholism is a multimodal problem, a variety of care providers with different, well-developed skills is required to meet the needs of diverse client populations. The quality of the client–health care provider relationship is a major factor. Alcoholic people need relationships with care providers who possess a sound knowledge of alcoholism and other health-related matters, a genuine interest in the client, and skills to provide the help needed.

The prognosis for recovery from alcoholism is no doubt related to the quality of care the client receives and is most likely based on more than the person's ability to remain abstinent. Prognosis from a nursing perspective is related to the client's ability to achieve a balance between the patterns of daily living and available resources. Nurses can provide the kind of environment needed to achieve stabilization of clients' health status and minimize factors that place them at risk. Nurses can instruct alcoholic persons concerning strategies to be employed in coping with activities and demands of daily life and assist them in using these strategies. Nurses can also facilitate the mobilization of internal resources and the use of available external resources.

Nurses work in a variety of settings and thus are uniquely placed to provide direct care to alcoholic people and their families. In every instance, appraisal is the initial step toward diagnosis and management planning. The role of the nurse in alcoholism is further explicated throughout this book.

REFERENCES

1. Armor, D. J., Polick, J. M., and Stambal, H. B.: Alcoholism and treatment, New York, 1978, John Wiley & Sons, Inc.
2. Cahalan, D.: Problem drinkers, San Francisco, 1970, Jossey-Bass, Inc., Publishers.
3. Carnevali, D. L., and Patrick, M.: Nursing management for the elderly, Philadelphia, 1979, J. B. Lippincott Co.
4. Davies, D. L.: Definitional issues in alcoholism. In Tarter, R. E., and Sugarman, A. A., editors: Alcoholism, Reading, Mass., 1976, Addison-Wesley Publishing Co., Inc.
5. Ewing, J. A., Rouse, B. A., and Pellizzari, E. D.: Alcohol sensitivity and ethnic background, American Journal of Psychiatry 131:206, 1974.
6. Goodwin, D. W., et al: Drinking problems in adopted and nonadopted sons of alcoholics, Archives of General Psychiatry 31:164, 1974.
7. Jellinek, E. M.: The disease concept of alcoholism, New Haven, Conn., 1960, The Hillhouse Press.
8. Keller, M.: The definition of alcoholism and the estimation of its prevalence In Pittman, D. J., et al., editors: Society, culture and drinking patterns, New York, 1962, John Wiley & Sons, Inc.
9. Little, D. E., and Carnevali, D. L.: Nursing care planning, Philadelphia, 1976, J. B. Lippincott Co.
10. Mann, M.: America's 150-year war: alcohol vs. alcoholism, Alcohol Health and Research World 1:5, Spring, 1973.
11. Marlatt, G. A., and Nathan, P. E.: Behavioral approaches to alcoholism, New Brunswick, N. J., 1978, Rutgers Center of Alcohol Studies.
12. Pattison, E. M.: Nonabstinent drinking goals in the treatment of alcoholism, Archives of General Psychiatry 33:923, 1976.
13. Plaut, T. F. A.: Alcohol problems: a report to the nation, New York, 1967, Oxford University Press.
14. Reinent, R. E.: The concept of alcoholism as a disease, Bulletin of the Menninger Clinic 32:21, 1968.

CHAPTER 2

Features of alcoholism

prevalence, definition, causation

Alcoholism is a complex phenomenon with differences in etiologic determinants and developmental processes. It is the purpose of this chapter to review the extent of the problem of alcoholism and to consider definitions as well as theories of causation. Such background information is essential, since it provides the conceptual base for carrying out accurate appraisal and formulating diagnoses. The depth and breadth of information gained during appraisal depend partly on the nurse's theoretic foundation.

PREVALENCE

An estimated 9.3 to 10 million persons in the adult population, or 7% of those 18 years of age or older, are alcoholics or problem drinkers.[18] Approximately 10% of adult men who drink are alcoholic, with the rates for women one third to one half of that number.[5, 18] Each of these persons affects three or four other people, including family, friends, and co-workers so that between 33 and 44 million people experience this problem at close hand.

Alcoholism ranks as this country's third greatest health problem.[11] As an example, about 30% of the admissions to state and county mental hospitals are given a primary diagnosis of alcohol problems. This increases to 50% for those in the 45- to 54-year age group. In addition, it is conservatively estimated that at any given time, 15% of the beds in a general hospital are filled with persons with alcohol-associated health problems, for example, gastritis or liver disease.[4]

Alcoholism is progressive and usually takes from five to twenty years to develop. Since it is not a single illness with a specific etiology, it is difficult to define.

DEFINITIONS

Since alcoholism seems to be the result of an interplay of many factors, there is no single definition. It is essential, however, to arrive at some common understanding about this phenomenon. It is important in deciding who should receive treatment; that is, should treatment be limited to individuals diagnosed as alcoholic according to a prevailing definition? It is important to the formulation of public policy; for example, definitions determine the direction of strategies in prevention and the policy toward treatment. In addition, it is important to the direction that research is likely to take; that is, studies of etiology are influenced by the way in which the definition is phrased.

One widely quoted definition was formulated by the World Health Organization, part of which follows:

Alcoholics are those excessive drinkers whose dependence on alcohol has attained such a degree it shows a noticeable mental disturbance or an interference with their bodily and mental health, their interpersonal relations and their smooth social and economic functioning, or who show the prodromal signs of such developments.[19]

Critics of this definition complain that it does not separate "harm" (mental disturbances and interferences with health and functioning) from dependence, nor does it acknowledge that these conditions can exist separately. One critic offers this alternative definition:

Alcoholism is intermittent or continual use of alcohol associated with dependency (psychological or physical) or harm in the sphere of mental, physical or social activity.[3]

However, this definition is still confusing and indicates the problem of defining alcoholism and differentiating it from patterns of alcohol use including heavy drinking. Harm associated with alcohol use can occur before dependency does, for example, in the case of someone who falls down the stairs and breaks an arm while intoxicated. If the person were generally a moderate social drinker and this was the first time in fifteen years of drinking that he had become intoxicated, it certainly could not be said that because he had experienced harm he was an alcoholic. *Repeated* harm seems essential to the definition of alcoholism and required for diagnosis.

In addition, psychologic dependence is usually distinguished from physical dependence. Psychologic dependence refers to feeling the need for a drink to cope, to relax, or to otherwise alter moods. For example, the person who comes home from a hard day's work shouting, "I need a drink," is manifesting psychologic dependence. Physical dependence, on the other hand, refers to an actual physiologic need for a drink. Classic components of physical dependence are an increasing tolerance for the effects of alcohol and appearance of a withdrawal syndrome when alcohol is removed from the body. Most experts would agree that a person exhibiting physical dependence is alcoholic. Psychologic dependence, however, usually occurs before and may never progress to physical dependence.

Alcoholism, then, occurs at one end of a continuum of drinking behaviors. Alcohol use may be light, moderate, or heavy; occasional or frequent.

Table 1. Criteria for the diagnosis of alcoholism*

Criterion	Diagnostic level
Major criteria	
Track I. Physiological and clinical	
A. Physiological dependency	
1. Physiological dependence as manifested by evidence of a *withdrawal syndrome*. When the intake of alcohol is interrupted or decreased without substitution of other sedation.† It must be remembered that overuse of other sedative drugs can produce a similar withdrawal state, which should be differentiated from withdrawal from alcohol.	
a. Gross tremor (differentiated from other causes of tremor)	1
b. Halluncinosis (differentiated from schizophrenic hallucinations or other psychoses)	1
c. Withdrawal seizures (differentiated from epilepsy and other seizure disorders)	1
d. Delirium tremens. Usually starts between the first and third day after withdrawal and minimally includes tremors, disorientation, and hallucinations	1
2. Evidence of *tolerance* to the effects of alcohol. (There may be a decrease in previously high levels of tolerance late in the course.) Although the degree of tolerance to alcohol in no way matches the degree of tolerance to other drugs, the behavioral effects of a given amount of alcohol vary greatly between alcoholic and nonalcoholic subjects.	
a. A blood alcohol level of more than 150 mg without gross evidence of intoxication	1
b. The consumption of one fifth of a gallon of whiskey or an equivalent amount of wine or beer daily, for more than 1 day, by a 180-lb individual	1
3. Alcoholic "blackout" periods. (Differential diagnosis from purely psychological fugue states and psychomotor seizures.)	
B. Clinical: Major alcohol-associated illnesses Alcoholism can be assumed to exist if major alcohol-associated illnesses develop in a person who drinks regularly. In such individuals evidence of physiological and psychological dependence should be searched for.	
Fatty degeneration in absence of other known cause	
Alcoholic hepatitis	2
Laennec's cirrhosis	1
Pancreatitis in the absence of cholelithiasis	2
Chronic gastritis	2
Hematological disorders:	3

*From Criteria Committee, National Council on Alcoholism: Criteria for the diagnosis of alcoholism, Annals of Internal Medicine **77**:249, 1972; American Journal of Psychiatry **129**:127, 1972.

†Some authorities term this "pharmacological addiction."

Table 1. Criteria for the diagnosis of alcoholism—cont'd

Criterion	Diagnostic level
Major criteria—cont'd	
Track I. *Physiological and clinical—cont'd*	
Anemia—hypochromic, normocytic, macrocytic, hemolytic with stomatocytosis, low folic acid	3
Clotting disorders—prothrombin elevation or thrombocytopenia	3
Wernicke-Korsakoff syndrome	2
Alcoholic cerebellar degeneration	1
Cerebral degeneration in absence of Alzheimer's disease or arteriosclerosis	2
Central pontine myelinolysis ⎫ Marchiafava-Bignami disease ⎬ diagnosis only possible postmortem	2
Peripheral neuropathy (*see* also beriberi)	2
Toxic amblyopia	3
Alcohol myopathy	2
Alcoholic cardiomyopathy	2
Beriberi	3
Pellagra	3

Track II. *Behavioral, psychological, and attitudinal*

All chronic conditions of psychological dependence occur in dynamic equilibrium with intrapsychic and interpersonal consequences. In alcoholism, similarly, there are varied effects on character and family. Like other chronic relapsing diseases, alcoholism produces vocational, social, and physical impairments. Therefore, the implications of these disruptions must be evaluated and related to the individual and his pattern of alcoholism. The following hehavior patterns show psychological dependence on alcohol in alcoholism.

1. Drinking despite strong medical contraindication known to patient	1
2. Drinking despite strong, identified social contraindication (job loss for intoxication, marriage disruption because of drinking, arrest for intoxication, driving while intoxicated)	1
3. Patient's subjective complaint of loss of control of alcohol consumption	2

Minor criteria
Track I. *Physiological and clinical*

A. Direct effects (ascertained by examination)	
1. Early	
Odor of alcohol on breath at time of medical appointment	2
2. Middle	
Alcoholic facies	2
Vascular engorgement of face	2
Toxic amblyopia	3
Increased incidence of infections	3

Continued.

Table 1. Criteria for the diagnosis of alcoholism—cont'd

Criterion	Diagnostic level
Minor criteria—cont'd	
Track I. *Physiological and clinical—cont'd*	
Cardiac arrhythmias	3
Peripheral neuropathy (*see* also Major criteria, Track I, B)	2
3. Late (*see* Major criteria, B)	
B. Indirect effects	
1. Early	
Tachycardia	3
Flushed face	3
Nocturnal diaphoresis	3
2. Middle	
Ecchymoses on lower extremities, arms, or chest	3
Cigarette or other burns on hands or chest	3
Hyperreflexia or, if drinking heavily, hyporeflexia (permanent hyporeflexia may be a residuum of alcoholic polyneuritis)	3
3. Late	
Decreased tolerance	3
C. Laboratory tests	
1. Direct	
Blood alcohol level at any time of more than 300 mg/100 ml or level of more than 100 mg/100 ml in routine examination	1
2. Indirect	
Serum osmolality (reflects blood alcohol levels): every 22.4 increase over 200 mOsm/liter reflects 50 mg/100 ml alcohol	2
Results of alcohol ingestion:	
Hypoglycemia	3
Hypochloremic alkalosis	3
Low magnesium level	2
Lactic acid elevation	3
Transient uric acid elevation	3
Potassium depletion	3
Indications of liver abnormality:	
SGPT* elevation	2
SGOT* elevation	3
BSP* elevation	2
Bilirubin elevation	2
Urinary urobilinogen elevation	2
Serum A/G* ratio reversal	2
Blood and blood clotting:	
Anemia—hypochromic, normocytic, macrocytic, hemolytic with stomatocytosis, low folic acid	3

*SGPT = serum glutamic-pyruvic transaminase; SGOT = serum glutamic-oxalacetic transaminase; BSP = sulfobromophthalein; A/G = albumin to globulin.

Table 1. Criteria for the diagnosis of alcoholism—cont'd

Criterion	Diagnostic level
Minor criteria—cont'd	
Track I. *Physiological and clinical—cont'd*	
Clotting disorders—prothrombin elevation, thrombocytopenia	3
ECG abnormalities:	
Cardiac arrhythmias: tachycardia: T waves dimpled, cloven, or spinous; atrial fibrillation, ventricular premature contractions: abnormal P waves	2
EEG abnormalities:	
Decreased or increased REM* sleep, depending on phase	3
Loss of delta sleep	3
Other reported findings	3
Decreased immune response	3
Decreased response to Synacthen test	3
Chromosomal damage from alcoholism	3
Track II. *Behavioral, psychological, and attitudinal*	
A. Behavioral	
1. Direct effects	
Early	
Gulping drinks	3
Surreptitious drinking	2
Morning drinking (assess nature of peer group behavior)	2
Middle	
Repeated conscious attempts at abstinence	2
Late	
Blatant indiscriminate use of alcohol	1
Skid Row or equivalent social level	2
2. Indirect effects	
Early	
Medical excuses from work for variety of reasons	2
Shifting from one alcoholic beverage to another	2
Preference for drinking companions, bars, and taverns	2
Loss of interest in activities not directly associated with drinking	2
Late	
Chooses employment that facilitates drinking	3
Frequent automobile accidents	3
History of family members undergoing psychiatric treatment; school and behavioral problems of children	3
Frequent change of residence for poorly defined reasons	3
Anxiety-relieving mechanisms, such as telephone calls inappropriate in time, distance, person, or motive (telephonitis)	2
Outbursts of rage and suicidal gestures while drinking	2

*REM = rapid eye movement.

Continued.

Table 1. Criteria for the diagnosis of alcoholism—cont'd

Criterion	Diagnostic level
Minor criteria—cont'd	
Track II. Behavioral, psychological, and attitudinal—cont'd	
B. Psychological and attitudinal	
1. Direct effects	
Early	
When talking freely, makes frequent reference to drinking alcohol, people being "bombed," "stoned," or admits drinking more than peer group	2
Middle	
Drinking to relieve anger, insomnia, fatigue, depression, social discomfort	2
Late	
Psychological symptoms consistent with permanent organic brain syndrome (*see* also Major criteria, Track I, B)	2
2. Indirect effects	
Early	
Unexplained changes in family, social, and business relationship: complaints about wife, job, and friends	3
Spouse makes complaints about drinking behavior, reported by patient or spouse	2
Major family disruptions; separation, divorce, threats of divorce	3
Job loss (owing to increasing interpersonal difficulties), frequent job changes, financial difficulties	3
Late	
Overt expression of more regressive defense mechanisms: denial, projection, and so on	3
Resentment, jealousy, paranoid attitudes	3
Symptoms of depression: isolation, crying, suicidal preoccupation	3
Feelings that he is "losing his mind"	2

Heavy, frequent drinking may become problematic and perhaps even develop into alcoholism. Alcoholism, by definition, refers to problems associated with drinking, but the reverse may not be the case. Some persons experience problems with drinking such as family conflict or inefficiency at work and alter their drinking patterns as a result so that their drinking does not become a problem for them again. Similarly, alcoholism requires alcohol use, but the reverse is not required; alcohol use may lead to alcoholism or it may not.

Perhaps the most far-reaching efforts in defining alcoholism are evident in the formulation of the "Criteria for the Diagnosis of Alcoholism" by members of a Committee of the American Medical Society on Alcoholism of the National Council on Alcoholism. These criteria, established as guidelines for diagnosis, are weighted for diagnostic significance and assembled according to type, "Physiological and Clinical" (Track I) and "Behavioral, Psychological, and Attitudinal" (Track II)[2] (Table 1). Each track is divided into major and minor criteria for diagnosis. Their relative importance to diagnosis is indicated by diagnostic levels. Diagnostic level 1 indicates a definite, level 2 indicates a probable, and level 3 indicates a potential diagnosis of alcoholism.

It is sufficient for the diagnosis if one or more of the major criteria are satisfied or if several of the minor criteria in Tracks I and II are present. These criteria must all be at diagnostic level 1, definite, to indicate alcoholism. Careful scrutiny is required to grasp the full meaning of these useful criteria.

When employed in nursing appraisal, diagnostic levels 2 and 3, probable and potential alcoholism, can be a means of early detection of alcoholism. Early discovery of alcoholism in a client can also be enhanced by the application of knowledge of theories of causation.

THEORIES OF CAUSATION

The occurrence of alcoholism in any one individual seems to result from numerous factors, since there is at present no known cause of alcoholism. Some evidence exists that numbers of persons affected by alcoholism increase proportionately in relation to the overall social consumption of alcohol.[13] In addition, personal characteristics such as genetic susceptibility as well as psychosocial and cultural factors make some persons more vulnerable to the development of alcoholism than others. Alcoholism has been called a psychosomatic condition to describe the subtle and constantly recurring interaction between the physiologic and psychologic components.[9] Some of these factors will be further outlined in the following material.

Genetic factors

It has long been recognized that alcoholism runs in families, but how much of this is the result of genetic as opposed to psychosocial and cultural factors is not certain. The results of one study of adopted children indicated that children of alcoholics are more likely to have alcohol problems in adulthood than children of nonalcoholics, despite being separated from their alcoholic parents in early life.[6] Being reared by an alcoholic parent figure or suffering a broken home by either death or separation of the adoptive parent did not seem to contribute to the final development of alcoholism. That is, persons who experienced such events were no more likely to develop alcoholism than those who did not. Adoptees were compared with their brothers who were not adopted.[7] The length of exposure to alcoholism in the parent was unrelated to the final development of alcoholism, but the severity in the parent predicted the occurrence of alcoholism in either the sons reared apart or in those reared by the alcoholic parent. The more severe the parental alcoholism, the greater the likelihood of a child's becoming alcoholic. The genetic theory, then, seems plausible and needs to be investigated further.[14]

A remaining question is whether an actual gene transmits the tendency to alcoholism or whether alcoholism is merely correlated with other inherited factors. Some of the questions raised about the latter have been whether metabolites of alcohol vary in some persons or whether some persons are, because of genetic makeup, more susceptible to the addicting effects.

Whatever the final answer on the genetic basis of alcoholism, psychosocial and cultural factors most likely also contribute to the causation of alcohol problems. After all, some children with alcoholic parents do not become alcoholics and others with no family history of alcoholism do, suggesting that other factors contribute to the development of alcoholism.

Psychosocial factors
Transactional theory

Proponents of the transactional theory believe that it is not the direct effects of alcohol on the individual which are reinforcing, as held by learning theorists, but rather the effects or consequences of being drunk. Alcoholism is seen as a style of interaction in which the individual and his family use drunkenness and helplessness as an excuse for responsibility-avoiding behavior.[8, 16] The following example illustrates the use of intoxication and helplessness to avoid responsibility.

A nurse visited a family with an alcoholic member. The husband-father functioned responsibly outside the home at his job but relinquished all responsibility on coming home each evening. He drank to the point of drunkenness and offered no physical or emotional support to his wife or children. His wife inadvertently reinforced this behavior by taking care of his physical needs, that is, cajoling food into him as he professed he was not hungry, cleaning up after him, and carefully tucking him into bed each night. A vicious circle had developed in which the wife ended up solidifying the behavior she wanted so desperately to change. When she could no longer cope with the demands placed on her, she sought professional help. As her reactions to her husband's drunkenness changed, he was able to discover the need to change also and eventually achieved sobriety. This example demonstrates that to effect change, all family members, not just the alcoholic person, must alter their interaction styles.[8]

Transactional theory also applies to individuals without families. Any person closely involved with the lone alcoholic, including health care providers or other workers in clinics, social agencies, or jails, can interact with him in such a way as to reinforce the alcoholism. Since it is the drunkenness that results in the social contact, it is the drinking behavior that gets reinforced.

Personality theory

A variety of personality attributes have been associated with alcoholism, but no single type is seen in all alcoholic persons and their role in causation is unclear. Personality theories of alcoholism are criticized for this lack of evidence. Some of the diverse personality traits suggested as causative factors in alcoholism are presented. For example, one fourth of alcoholic men develop alcoholism as part of an antisocial personality.[15] Alcoholic women experience a greater amount of depression than men but whether this condition precedes the alcoholism is not always clear. Also associated with excessive use of alcohol are heightened anxiety, low self-esteem, dependency, poor impulse control, low frustration tolerance, and lack of power.[1] In the latter instance, the alcoholic person is viewed as needing to feel power that does not exist in reality and so uses alcohol for an initial uplift and to permit fantasies of importance. The example of the alcoholic husband described earlier could fit into the dependency model, since it could be said that he has a need to be taken care of or to feel dependent in at least some aspect of his life. Whether personality attributes associated with alcoholism occur prior to or after its development is not certain.

Longitudinal studies are needed to solve the problem of cause and effect. The premorbid personality of the alcoholic person has been inferred from theoretic analyses of personality makeup once alcoholism is established. This practice sheds no light on those attributes present when heavy drinking is initiated.

Social factors

The presence of alcoholism in a community has been hypothetically correlated with a degree of social stress. In this framework the more that people experience social deprivation, such as poor housing and discrimination, the more likely they are to consume alcohol excessively in response. Associated with this is the degree to which the society offers alternatives to the release of tension and provides substitute means of satisfaction. A society that offers few alternatives to drinking as a tension releaser will have a high rate of alcoholism. The consumption of alcohol then takes precedence over alternate ways to handle life problems.[10]

In addition to feelings of tension, adverse economic and psychosocial conditions may result in persons becoming alienated from the society in which they live and rejecting its norms. Anomy, the condition of normlessness, has been implicated in the development of alcoholism.[12] The more severe the alcoholism, the greater the anomy, which then perpetuates alcoholic drinking.

Another social factor that may play a role in the development of excessive drinking or alcoholism is advertising. The reasoning is as follows: If advertisers are successful in increasing overall consumption, then the rate of alcoholism is also raised. If advertising encourages more people to drink, a percentage of whom become alcoholic, then alcoholism has increased as an indirect result of advertising. Research needs to determine what, if any, relationship does actually exist between these variables.

Cultural factors

Culturally derived explanations have been sought for the greatly varying rates of alcoholism among different cultural groups. Italians and Jews, for example, traditionally have had low rates of alcoholism. Speculation as to reasons include the following observations. In groups showing low alcoholism rates, the use of alcohol is circumscribed and associated with meals. Drinking is taken for granted and given no special significance. No positive value is associated with amounts consumed, and drunkenness is discouraged.[17] In addition, children partake of small amounts of alcoholic beverages served with meals, and thus drinking is not seen as solely an adult behavior. All of these factors probably contribute to low rates of alcoholism in these cultures but are not necessary and sufficient conditions to explain varying rates.

The French, on the other hand, have high rates of alcoholism along with patterns similar to those just described. Although alcohol is consumed with meals and by young people, drunkenness is not seen as problematic. Whether it is this attitude toward drinking behavior that is associated with the development of alcoholism is not yet known.

Although the study of different cultures' attitudes toward and use of alcohol may be enlightening, it is unclear what effects it might have in altering rates of alcoholism. What works in one culture to mitigate alcoholism may fail when transposed to another cultural group. Cultural variation exists in the United States and shapes drinking patterns within the larger society. Thus an individual may have cultural patterns of drinking because of being Jewish or Italian, for example, in addition to having certain patterns of drinking because of being American.

REFERENCES

1. Blane, H.: The personality of the alcoholic, New York, 1968, Harper & Row, Publishers.
2. Criteria Committee, National Council on Alcoholism: Criteria for the diagnosis of alcoholism, Annals of Internal Med, **77**:249, 1972; American Journal of Psychiatry 129:127-135, 1972.

3. Davies, D. L.: Definitional issues in alcoholism. In Tarter, R. E., and Sugarman, A. A., editors: Alcoholism, Reading, Mass., 1976, Addison-Wesley Publishing Co., Inc.
4. Diagnostic distribution of admissions to inpatient services of state and county mental hospitals, Mental Health Statistical Note No. 138, Rockville, Md., 1975, National Institute of Mental Health.
5. Estes, N. J., and Heinemann, M. E.: Perspectives on alcoholism. In Longo, D., and Williams, R. A., editors: Contemporary clinical practice in psychosocial nursing: assessment and intervention, New York, 1978, Appleton-Century-Crofts.
6. Goodwin, D. W., et al.: Alcohol problems in adoptees raised apart from alcoholic biological parents, Archives of General Psychiatry **28**:238, 1973.
7. Goodwin, D. W., et al.: Drinking problems in adopted and nonadopted sons of alcoholics, Archives of General Psychiatry **31**:164, 1974.
8. Gorad, S. L., McCourt, W. F., and Cobb, J. C.: A communications approach to alcoholism, Quarterly Journal of Studies on Alcohol **32**:651, 1971.
9. Hershon, H.: Learning to be an alcoholic, Journal of Psychosomatic Research **21**:297, 1977.
10. Marlatt, G. A., and Nathan, P. E.: Behavioral approaches to alcoholism, New Brunswick, N.J., 1978, Rutgers Center of Alcohol Studies.
11. Noble, E. P.: Foreward. In Birnbaum, I., and Parker, E. S., editors: Alcohol and human memory, New York, 1977, John Wiley & Sons, Inc.
12. Phillips, L. A.: An application of anomy theory to the study of alcoholism, Journal of Studies on Alcohol **37**:78, 1976.
13. Popham, R. E., et al.: The effectiveness of legal measure in the prevention of alcohol problems, Addictive Diseases **2**:497, 1976.
14. Schuckit, M. A.: A half-sibling study of alcoholism: some reflections. In Pasamanick, B., editor: Compendium of work receiving the Hofheimer Award. In press.
15. Schuckit, M. A.: Alcoholism and sociopathy—diagnostic confusion, Quarterly Journal of Studies on Alcohol **34**:157, 1973.
16. Steiner, C.: Games alcoholics play, New York, 1971, Grover Press.
17. United States Department of Health, Education, and Welfare, Alcohol and health, Vol. 2, Washington, D.C., 1974, U. S. Government Printing Office.
18. United States Department of Health, Education and Welfare, Alcohol and health, Vol. 3, Washington, D.C., 1978, U.S. Government Printing Office.
19. Expert Committee on Mental Health, First Report of the Alcoholism Subcommittee, WHO Technical Report Series no. 42, Geneva, 1951, World Health Organization.

CHAPTER 3

Features of alcoholism

physiologic and psychosocial aspects

Alcoholic persons differ in the responses they exhibit to excessive alcohol consumption and to the consequences they experience as a result of long-term consumption. Alcohol-associated physiologic and psychosocial deviations for which the alcoholic person is at risk are described in this chapter.

PHYSIOLOGIC ASPECTS

Both short- and long-term alcohol consumption affects almost every organ system in the body. Alcohol metabolism, intoxication, tolerance to and physical dependence on alcohol, as well as the physiologic concomitants of chronic consumption on various body systems, will be described.

Metabolism

In nonaddicted individuals alcohol is metabolized in a zero-order kinetic way; that is, a fixed amount of alcohol is metabolized in a specific period of time. Generally, an ounce of whiskey, approximately a 5-ounce glass of wine, or a 12-ounce bottle of beer are about equivalent. Thus 4 ounces of whiskey are about equivalent to four glasses of wine or four bottles of beer.

Alcohol is metabolized almost exclusively in the liver by means of three possible pathways. The *alcohol dehydrogenase* (ADH) system is the main pathway for alcohol metabolism and ultimately converts alcohol into carbon dioxide and water (Fig. 2). Another system that mediates the metabolism of alcohol is the *microsomal ethanol oxidizing system* (MEOS). MEOS activity is stimulated by exposure to alcohol. This pathway becomes increasingly important to alcoholic persons who frequently ingest large amounts of alcohol. Largely because of activation of the MEOS, alcoholics metabolize alcohol in a first-order kinetic way; that is, the greater the blood alcohol concentration, the faster the metabolism.[12] *Catalase* is a third, but relatively insignificant, mechanism for metabolizing ethanol.

The transfer of hydrogen to nicotinamide-adenine-dinucleotide (NAD), which occurs during metabolism, alters the NADH/NAD ratio and is responsible for a number of metabolic abnormalities. These include reduced glu-

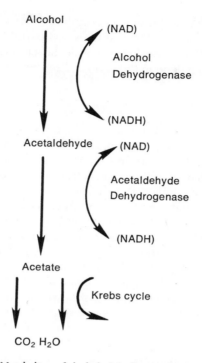

Fig. 2. Metabolism of alcohol: dehydrogenase pathway.

coneogenesis, which leads to hypoglycemia. Another abnormality is hyperlactacidemia, which contributes to acidosis and reduces the capacity of the kidney to excrete uric acid, leading in turn to hyperuricemia and symptoms of gout. In addition, the increased NADH/NAD ratio leads to accumulation of hepatic triglycerides because of the promotion of synthesis and trapping of fatty acids.[17] At the same time the oxidation of these fatty acids by the liver is decreased in preference for alcohol. Thus fat accumulates throughout the body, especially in the liver and muscles.

Also toxic to body tissues and implicated in alcohol-associated physiologic sequelae is acetaldehyde, the first by-product of alcohol metabolism. Acetaldehyde seems to be involved in a number of the aberrant effects associated with both acute and chronic alcohol use. Nothing definitive can be said about this relationship, however, since it depends on the concentration of acetaldehyde at the site of action with a particular dose of alcohol. Acetaldehyde assay methods show that levels are low after alcohol consumption, but such methods need to be improved.[18] Although alcoholic persons seem to exhibit slightly higher levels of acetaldehyde than normal, grossly elevated levels are seen currently only in the presence of disulfiram (Antabuse) and other alcohol-sensitizing compounds. More studies comparing the concentration of acetaldehyde with the observed effects of alcohol are needed to delineate the role played by acetaldehyde in the various disorders for which alcoholic persons are at risk.[18]

Intoxication

If alcohol is consumed at the rate in which it can be metabolized, that is, 0.5 ounce of absolute alcohol an hour, it will be almost imperceptible in the blood. Blood alcohol levels rise in proportion to the amount of alcohol consumed per hour. Alcohol in the blood is transported to all tissues, including the nerves, and it is the effect of alcohol on the nervous system that results in the observable signs and symptoms of intoxication. The behavioral effects of alcohol in a nonalcoholic person at various blood levels are shown in Table 2.

Effects exhibited depend on the concentration of alcohol in the blood, which in turn depends on the rapidity with which *alcohol is absorbed from the stomach and upper part of the small intestine,* as well as on the weight and sex of the drinking individual. Alcohol is absorbed more quickly from an empty stomach and when combined with carbonated beverages. The latter seems to be because the carbonation results in a more rapid diffusion of alcohol across the cell membrane and into the bloodstream. Generally, heavier individuals can consume more than lighter individuals because they have an increased total body water in which to dilute the alcohol. This is less true, however, if all the weight is fat. Since women have a higher proportion of body fat, and thus less total body water pound for pound than men, they usually can consume less alcohol than a similarly sized man and still achieve like effects.

Tolerance and physical dependence

Another factor influencing behavior after consumption of alcohol is the phenomenon of tolerance. Tolerance refers to the biologic adaptation that nerve cells undergo in response to prolonged exposure to high blood alcohol levels. Repeated alcohol consumption eventually results in a diminished response. Evidence of tolerance consists of a need to increase the amount of alcohol consumed to produce specific effects. Thus a person who regularly consumes alcohol gradually needs to consume more and more alcohol on each drinking occasion to achieve an associated "high." When behavior is much less affected than would be expected by the blood alcohol levels, tolerance can be inferred. An intoxicated person involved in a car accident was observed in an urban emergency room. Her affect was jocular, her speech was slurred, and she was staggering a bit. A blood alcohol level determination showed that the concentration of alcohol in her blood was 0.40%. As can

Table 2. Alcohol ingestion and alcohol blood levels*†

Amount of alcohol ingested	Percent of alcohol in blood	Symptoms
2 ounces of whiskey	0.05%	Not under the influence, appear normal
4 ounces of whiskey	0.10% (common legal limit for operation of motor vehicle)	Beginning of outward physical symptoms: Emotional lability (boastfulness, exhilaration, talkativeness, remorse, belligerence) Slight muscular incoordination, such as slowed reaction time, ataxia Decreased inhibitions
6 ounces of whiskey	0.15%	"Under the influence": Sensory disturbances (decreased pain sense, diplopia, vertigo, slurred speech) Confusion Staggering gait Rapid pulse Diaphoresis
8 ounces of whiskey (½ pint)	0.20%	"Acutely intoxicated": Marked decrease in response to stimuli Muscular incoordination approaching paralysis Nausea and vomiting Drowsiness and/or stupor
	0.30-0.40%	Symptoms listed for 0.15% Complete unconsciousness Impaired or absent tendon reflexes Peripheral vascular collapse (hypotension, tachycardia, cold pale skin, hypothermia, slow stertorous respiration) Seizures (if present may also indicate hypoglycemia)
1½-2 pints whiskey	0.50%	Death due to cardiac or respiratory arrest or aspiration pneumonitis

*From Ansbaugh, P.: Emergency management of intoxicated patients with head injuries, Journal of Emergency nursing 3:10, May/June, 1977.
†The blood levels are the *minimum* that occur in an average (160-pound) adult 30 to 45 minutes after ingestion.

be seen in Table 2, complete unconsciousness could have been expected, not just the relatively minor symptoms just described. This is an example of tolerance.

Also associated with central nervous system adaptation to repeated alcohol exposure is physical dependence, which can be said to have developed if sudden cessation of drinking causes specific physiologic and behavioral changes. These changes are referred to as the withdrawal syndrome.

Tolerance and physical dependence do not necessarily develop in conjunction with each other and may develop by different mechanisms.[18] There is speculation that the mechanisms of tolerance and physical dependence may occur because of either some alcohol effect on neurotransmitters or genetic variances in transmitters or receptor complexes. A compensatory increase in the amount of acetylcholine, 5-hydroxytryptamine, N-adrenaline, and other neurotransmitters available in the synaptic clefts may occur with repeated alcohol consumption.[13] Until the molecular basis of these possible changes is elucidated, such suggestions are highly conjectural.

Withdrawal

Symptoms of alcohol withdrawal appear when consumption stops completely or is decreased. Thus withdrawal reactions can begin before all the alcohol has been eliminated from the body. As an alcoholic person's blood

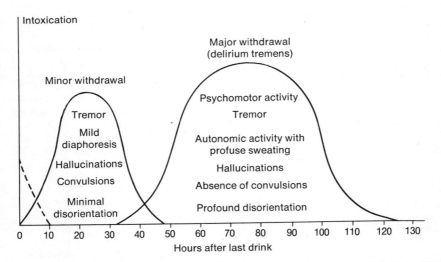

Fig. 3. Clinical findings during the minor (early) alcohol withdrawal syndrome and the major withdrawal syndrome (delirium tremens). (From Wolfe, S. M., and Victor, M.: In Mello, N. K., and Mendelson, J. H., editors: Recent advances in studies of alcoholism, Rockville, Md., 1970, National Institute of Alcohol and Alcoholism.)

alcohol level falls, the central and autonomic nervous systems, which have adapted to alcohol's sedative effect, become overactive.[31] According to the neurotransmitter hypothesis described earlier, decreasing blood alcohol levels result in a decompensated system with an excess availability of synaptic neurotransmitters. This produces neuronal hyperexcitability of graded intensity that ranges from mild tremor, tachycardia and hypertension, diaphoresis, and insomnia, to grand mal seizures, hallucinations, and disorientation.[13] The characteristic progression of different components of the syndrome can be seen in Fig. 3.[35] The tremor begins early; generalized tonic-clonic seizures and relatively benign kinds of hallucinations may begin at about 24 hours after cessation of drinking. The most severe abnormality, delirium tremens, does not begin until 3 to 5 days later. Both the intensity and advancement of the symptoms, as well as the time of onset, can be predicted. This aspect of withdrawal will be discussed further in Chapter 6.

Alcohol's effect on various body systems

As mentioned previously, when alcohol is consumed faster than it can be metabolized, it accumulates in the bloodstream and thereby reaches every cell in the body. In addition, tolerance allows for large amounts to be accumulated. As a result, the physiologic effects of excessive alcohol consumption are extensive. Alcohol adversely affects nearly every body system, with some systems being more affected than others. The specific system and personal differences as well as the amount and length of alcohol consumption all play a part in determining the risk of deleterious consequences.

Gastrointestinal system

Since functions associated with the gastrointestinal tract begin in the mouth and end at the rectum, this framework will serve discussion purposes of this section. Alcohol irritates the gastrointestinal system, which can be crudely observed when a person consumes alcohol. Depending on the beverage, alcohol to greater or lesser degrees "burns" the mouth and throat as it is drunk and swallowed. Even though it cannot be felt, this irritant effect continues throughout the gastrointestinal tract and inflammation and local injury resulting in bleeding and malabsorption can occur at any point in the system.

Mouth and throat. Excessive consumption has been associated with an increased incidence of cancer in general and oral cancer in particular.[28] The explanation for this is clouded by the fact that a vast proportion of excessive drinkers also smoke, and smoking by itself increases the risks of developing head and neck cancer. However, these risks seem to be even greater with alcohol consumption. The best explanation for the present time is that alcohol and smoking probably act synergistically, resulting in an increased incidence of cancer.

Esophagus. Esophagitis can occur because of the irritating, inflammatory effects of alcohol and also as a result of vomiting, which is often associated with alcohol abuse. Frequent, severe vomiting may lead to a Mallory-Weiss or Boerhaave syndrome. The Mallory-Weiss syndrome refers to a mucosal laceration that can occur across the gastroesophageal junction. This condition is usually painless, but if hematemesis occurs in a patient, a Mallory-Weiss tear should be suspected and evaluated further by endoscopy. The hemorrhage is usually self-limited if the vomiting can be controlled.

The Boerhaave syndrome, on the other hand, is exquisitely painful. This frank rupture of the lower esophagus may occur associated with coughing, lifting, or having a seizure, besides vomiting.[7] It is the leakage of gastric contents into the chest cavity that causes the severe pain and usually leads to death.

The esophagus is also adversely affected as a consequence of the liver damage seen in some alcoholic persons. Esophageal varices result from defective blood flow through the liver. As the pressure in these vessels increases, they may rupture, resulting in hemorrhage and sometimes death. It was once thought that most gastrointestinal hemorrhages occurring in alcoholic persons were secondary to gastric or duodenal ulcers. Recent evidence suggests that esophageal varices and Mallory-Weiss tears outrank ulcers as the causes of gastrointestinal hemorrhages in alcoholic persons.[11]

Stomach. As mentioned, ulcers are not the major cause of gastrointestinal bleeding in alcoholic persons, nor are they even as common an occurrence as once believed.[7] The most common sequela to alcohol abuse affecting the stomach is erosive gastritis. Epigastric distress, nausea, vomiting, and distention mark this syndrome, which is caused by alcohol's disruption of the stomach's protective mucosal cell barrier. When intact, this barrier prevents autodigestion of the stomach by the hydrochloric acid it secretes. When disrupted, stomach cells as well as blood vessels can be eroded and bleed. Since aspirin has a similar effect, only well-buffered aspirin or aspirin substitutes should be given to alcoholic persons.

Intestines. Alcohol's irritant, inflammatory effects on the small intestine can result in enteritis and the malabsorption of a number of different substances, including essential nutrients from food.[19] Thus even seemingly well-fed excessive drinkers may exhibit signs and symptoms of nutritional deficiencies.

Colitis and hemorrhoids are the two alcohol-associated effects on the large intestine. Again, colitis is caused by alcohol's irritant effects, whereas hemorrhoids occur secondarily to the impaired blood flow of portal hypertension.

Liver. The liver is highly susceptible to the effects of alcohol because it is the primary site of alcohol metabolism. There seems to be a relationship

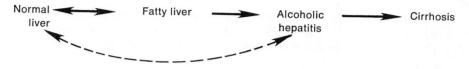

Fig. 4. Progression of liver disease in alcoholic persons.

between the severity of liver disease and the duration and amount of excessive alcohol consumption. The longer and more continuous the drinking, the greater the risk of harm to the liver. Excessive alcohol consumption can cause fatty liver, alcoholic hepatitis, or cirrhosis. These disorders can exist singly or in combination and often occur in progression (Fig. 4).

ALCOHOLIC FATTY LIVER. As mentioned earlier, one of the metabolic abnormalities that results from the metabolism of alcohol is the accumulation of free fatty acids, causing increased concentrations of fat within the liver cell. Even modest doses of alcohol, with resultant blood levels well below the point of intoxication, regularly produce increased fat concentrations.[7]

Clinical manifestations of fatty liver in the alcoholic are usually minor and consist of liver enlargement and minimal derangements in liver function tests. Rarely, but especially in "binge" drinkers, fatty liver may become acute and severe symptoms such as abdominal pain, anorexia, and jaundice may occur.[7] Most often fatty liver is completely reversible with abstinence from alcohol.

ALCOHOLIC HEPATITIS. In some persons, continued heavy drinking results in alcoholic hepatitis, a syndrome of necrosis and inflammation that can be a serious, life-threatening condition. Loss of liver substance and scarring (fibrosis) occur, a process that may develop insidiously and gradually over many months or years or rapidly in the course of a few weeks. Clinical manifestations include hepatomegaly, jaundice, hepatic pain, fever, leukocytosis, and sometimes ascites.[7]

The reversibility of alcoholic hepatitis is variable and depends on its severity and chronicity.[7] When damage reaches a stage of irreversible distortion of hepatic structure, neither abstinence nor continuation of drinking deters further development of the disease, and cirrhosis is the result.

ALCOHOLIC CIRRHOSIS. Cirrhosis is advanced necrosis with resultant scarring associated with the formation of nodules, both of which serve to distort the normal architecture of the liver. The cirrhotic process, with distortion and obliteration of the normal liver lobules, is generally irreversible even with abstinence from alcohol.[7] In addition to the signs and symptoms associated with hepatitis, the cirrhotic patient is likely to develop portal hypertension with ascites and/or edema as well as increased shunting of portal blood around the liver. Esophageal varices and encephalopathy are the end results of these physiologic processes.[7]

It was recently thought that much of the liver damage caused by alcoholism was the result of the nutritional deficiencies found in most alcoholic persons. It is now known that alcohol has a direct toxic effect on the liver independent of diet. A poor diet may enhance debilitation, of course, just like an adequate diet enhances recovery. But only abstinence from alcohol will cause any significant change in the course of alcoholic liver disease.

Pancreas. Another physiologic abnormality associated with excessive alcohol consumption is pancreatitis. Approximately one half of all cases of pancreatitis are alcohol related.[33] Single, initial episodes are described as "acute" and repeated episodes as "chronic."

ACUTE ALCOHOLIC PANCREATITIS. This condition is most often seen in men of 25 to 65 years of age who have been drinking heavily for five to ten years or more. Although there may be no characteristic clinical picture, the outstanding symptom is severe, constant epigastric pain, which frequently radiates to the back. Nausea and vomiting are common. The patient usually looks ill, and there may be signs of abdominal tenderness and distention. The hallmark of this syndrome is the relationship of onset of symptoms to alcohol ingestion. They usually begin 1 or 2 days after a drinking bout.

CHRONIC ALCOHOLIC PANCREATITIS. The onset of this illness is often insidious. The associated pain is chronic and may lead to analgesic abuse and narcotic addiction. Besides pain, manifestations of this condition include exocrine insufficiency (fat malabsorption leading to weight loss, malnutrition, foul-smelling, bulky stools often with diarrhea) and endocrine insufficiency (diabetes mellitus).[7]

Although the mechanisms by which acute and chronic pancreatitis may develop are still being debated, recent thought is that chronic, heavy alcohol ingestion has direct, toxic effects on the pancreas.[7] Thus abstinence from alcohol is implicated in treatment of these conditions.

Neurologic system

In addition to the manifestations of intoxication and withdrawal, alcohol has other deleterious effects on both the central and peripheral nervous systems. Acute alcohol-associated injury to the nervous system can occur as a result of trauma, for example, subdural hematoma. In addition, the fact that chronic exposure to alcohol leads to brain damage has been known and accepted for a long time even by the general public. Short-term memory loss, one form of which is blackouts, is a fairly common concomitant to intoxication due to excessive alcohol consumption. Blackouts are periods of amnesia that occur when a person is intoxicated. The individual can function without obvious impairment but cannot remember some, or all, of his activities the next day or when sober. The exact mechanism by which alcohol-associated brain impairment occurs is not known. Nutritional deficiencies have been implicated in the development of the Wernicke-Korsakoff syndrome and peripheral polyneuropathies. Intravascular agglutination (sludging), which results in cellular hypoxia, has been suggested as the cause of chronic brain damage. Sludging, with resultant cell destruction due to hypoxia, occurs each time a person is intoxicated. With repeated bouts of intoxication more and more cells die, eventually resulting in clinically obvious impairment. The various alcohol-associated nervous system disorders will be considered separately.

Sleep disturbances. Alcohol adversely affects sleep patterns, resulting in frequent awakening, restless sleeps, insomnia, and night terrors.[27] Alcohol, like other sedative hypnotic drugs, tends to suppress the amount of rapid eye movement (REM) or dreaming sleep obtained during a normal night's sleep. REM sleep deprivation impairs concentration and memory and causes anxiety, tiredness, and irritability.[28] When alcohol consumption stops, REM rebound occurs and the person spends more time at this stage than usual. In addition, it seems that alcoholic persons essentially have no stage 4, or deep, sleep, whether they are drinking or not. Stage 3 sleep diminishes while the individual is drinking but then recovers. Sleep stages 3 and 4 comprise what is known as slow-wave sleep, which is also essential to healthy functioning.[27] Sleep stages 1 and 2 seem to be unaffected by alcohol consumption.

The reason why alcohol interferes with certain phases of normal sleep is not yet known. It has been noted that the sleep patterns of alcoholic people are usually similar to those of nonalcoholic persons who are much older. The suggestion is that alcohol accelerates the normal aging of the brain, thereby disrupting sleep. Another hypothesis is that alcohol affects biogenic amines, which in turn are required for sleep.

Peripheral neuropathy. The cause of peripheral neuropathies found in alcoholic persons is a deficiency of B vitamins, especially thiamine. The development of clinical manifestations is usually slow, extending over a period of weeks or months. Involvement is bilateral and symmetric, beginning distally and occurring in the feet before the hands. Sensory manifestations such as numbness, pain, paresthesias (burning, prickling, tingling), and hyperesthesias on pressure occur first and are usually followed by motor involvement such as weakness, muscle atrophy, footdrop, and ataxic gait.[8] These symptoms appear in a characteristic "stocking-glove" fashion, that is, in the locale that would be covered by stockings on the feet or gloves on the hands. Vibratory and position sense and reflexes become impaired.

Wernicke-Korsakoff syndrome. What used to be considered two separate entities, Wernicke's encephalopathy and Korsakoff's psychosis, are now generally considered to be a single entity, since they most frequently occur in conjunction with each other. In addition, both seem to be caused by the same mechanism, a deficiency in thiamine (vitamin B_1).

Vitamin deficiencies in general are common in alcoholics because their food intake is usually decreased and what is ingested tends to be malabsorbed. In addition to these factors, thiamine, to be bioavailable, must be phosphorylated in the liver. Since liver function is impaired in many alcoholic persons, thiamine deficiency may occur because it cannot be converted to a metabolically active form. Thiamine activates the tricarboxylic acid (Krebs) cycle, which is the primary source of energy for nerve cells. Thus if not enough thiamine is available, nerve cell functioning is impaired. *It is important for nurses to know that carbohydrate metabolism increases the demand for thiamine; consequently, intravenous glucose administration may precipitate Wernicke-Korsakoff syndrome in patients with marginal thiamine levels.*[27] In such patients the addition of thiamine to intravenous solutions is essential. In fact, short-term (up to 5 days) prophylactic administration of thiamine to known or suspected alcoholic persons has become a routine treatment approach.

The typical patient with Wernicke-Korsakoff syndrome is a chronic alcoholic of 40 to 60 years of age who becomes confused and excited. Peripheral neuropathy is most often present in conjunction with this syndrome. After a few days to several weeks, diplopia, the first real diagnostic clue, develops secondarily to a third or sixth cranial nerve palsy.[27]

The mental picture is one of severe recent memory loss, a loss of capacity for introspection and judgment of what might be true or plausible, and an apparent urge to "cover up" the memory deficit with stories that may be obviously untrue or absurd.[27] Disturbances of mood and affect suggestive of dementia may occur in later stages. Once the patient has progressed to this stage, lifetime custodial care may be the only treatment option.

Organic brain syndrome. Also known as dementia, organic brain syndrome is associated with a diffuse loss of functioning brain tissue and may have a number of causes including alcoholism.[27] Personality changes such as irritability, social withdrawal, inconsiderateness, petulance, or moral laxity are common. As the syndrome worsens, confusion, disorientation, and recent memory deficit are noticed.[27] General forgetfulness and poor judgment are classic. Further deterioration of brain tissue leads to the affected individual losing all control of his person and surroundings and requiring custodial care.

Degenerative syndromes. *Cerebellar degeneration* is clinically manifested by the gradual development of ataxic gait; incoordination, spasticity, and tremors of arms and legs; nystagmus; and dysarthria in which the speech is thick and the gait is broad based and halting.[8] There are two speculations as to cause: that it either is due to a vitamin deficiency or to the chronic exposure of cerebellar cells to toxic levels of acetaldehyde. The typical patient is a chronic alcoholic person over 50 years of age, usually male, who has neglected nutrition. At this late stage of body damage secondary to alcoholism, some residual permanent damage is to be expected even if abstinence is now achieved.

Degeneration of the corpus callosum (Marchiafava-Bignami disease) was discovered in Italians who drank crude red wine. It is a rare disease that occurs in older, chronic alcoholic persons and is characterized by behavioral problems such as confusion, excitement, dementia, and focal neurologic signs such as generalized tonic-clonic seizures, paresis, aphasia, and apraxia.[8, 27]

Central pontine myelinolysis, as with the other degenerative diseases, occurs in people whose alcoholism is of long duration. Clinically, there is an acute onset of quadriplegia and pseudobulbar palsy, manifested by nystagmus, slurred speech, impaired ocular convergence, dysphagia, paresis of the lower portion of the face with diminished cough and gag reflexes, and respiratory disturbances.[8, 27] No method of treatment is known, and most cases end fatally.

Alcoholic amblyopia. A relatively rare form of eye disorder occurs in chronic alcoholic persons and is usually associated with nutritional deficits. The patient experiences a painless, bilateral blurring of vision with reduced visual acuity and scotomas.[27] These symptoms occur over a period of several weeks to months. Improvement can be expected with dietary adjustment and vitamin supplements.

Alcoholic pellagra. An acute deficiency of niacin can occur in alcoholic persons as a result of malnutrition, malabsorption, or increased demand for niacin in the form of NAD. The symptoms consist of psychiatric disturbances, including confusion, depression, hallucinations, and delirium; dermatitis; and alimentary tract disorders, including glossitis, stomatitis, diarrhea, or constipation.[27] Treatment consists of replacement of niacin.

Cardiovascular system

Alcohol exerts a number of direct and indirect deleterious effects on the cardiovascular system and is in no way beneficial to persons with heart disease, as was once believed. With large doses of alcohol, the mechanical performance of the heart is decreased, which results in lessened cardiac output. Diminished output slows the entire circulatory system, resulting in an accumulation of lactic acid in the periphery, dilatation of the blood vessels, and a compensatory tachycardia. Other symptoms include shortness of breath, palpitations, decreased exercise tolerance, increased heart size, atrial fibrillation, excessive nocturnal diaphoresis, a narrow pulse pressure, intermittent paroxysmal nocturnal dyspnea, and edema.[32] As the condition worsens, congestive heart failure may occur.

Cardiac arrhythmias have been observed during weekend or holiday drinking episodes in persons with no prior history of heart disease.[6] The arrhythmias are associated with conduction delays and depressed cardiac performance indicative of early cardiomyopathy. This symptom picture has been termed the "holiday heart" syndrome.

Alcoholic cardiomyopathy is a long-term cardiac effect that usually occurs after many years of heavy drinking. A direct toxic effect of alcohol that results in triglyceride accumulation in, and altered permeability of, the cardiac cell is implicated in the etiology. The exact mechanism is unknown. Clinical findings are those of congestive heart failure, for example, tachycardia, orthopnea, and nonproductive cough.

Indirect cardiac effects occur secondarily to withdrawal from alcohol. Tachycardia and hypertension are common occurrences and place a heavy workload on the heart. A prolonged, severe detoxification may lead to an extreme state of fatigue and perhaps sudden death due to cardiogenic shock, cardiac standstill, ventricular fibrillation and flutter, or abrupt left-sided heart failure.[16]

Beriberi heart disease can occur and is due to thiamine deficiency. Significant reduction in peripheral vascular resistance is characteristic of the disease and leads to an increased cardiac output and decreased circulation time (the opposite symptoms of alcoholic cardiomyopathy). Thiamine replacement is essential to recovery.

Finally, alcohol causes peripheral blood vessels to dilate, which increases body heat loss. It may be essential to diminish heat loss before hypothermia occurs.

Respiratory system

Chronic, obstructive pulmonary disease occurs frequently in alcoholic persons. It seems to be due to the direct toxic effects of alcohol on pulmonary tissue, which results in an impaired clearance of bacteria and secretions from the lungs.[20] As a result, the lungs become more susceptible to bronchial infections and the injurious effects of cigarette smoking and air pollution. Once a certain degree of injury takes place, even abstinence from alcohol does not ensure return to normal.

Since most alcoholic people smoke, they are susceptible to a wide variety of respiratory problems, such as pneumonia. The incidence of tuberculosis is high. Alcohol suppresses the immune system so that the body has difficulty responding to and eliminating noxious agents.

Genitourinary system

The popular belief that alcohol is a diuretic is true only while the blood alcohol level rises and stabilizes. As it falls, an antidiuretic effect causes fluid retention.[2] As a result, alcoholic persons are more likely to be overhydrated than dehydrated, except in cases of vomiting and/or diarrhea.

Heavy alcohol consumption causes the kidney to excrete potassium and magnesium. Both hypokalemia and hypomagnesemia have implications for cardiac functioning. In addition, it has been suggested that hypomagnesemia is the causative factor in withdrawal seizures.

Hypogonadism, hypoandrogenization, and hyperestrogenization occur in chronic alcoholic men. Alcohol and acetaldehyde have a direct toxic effect on the testes, resulting in decreased plasma testosterone, decreased fertility, atrophic testes, and inadequate secondary sex characteristics. Clinically reduced beard growth, prostatic atrophy, reduced libido, and impotence are prominent findings.[29] On the other hand, estrogen-induced characteristics are acquired. The female physical characteristics known to occur in alcoholic men include gynecomastia, diminished body hair, and the accumulation of hypogastric and pelvic fat pads.[29] The development of spider angiomas may also be a physical sign of hyperestrogenization.

The effects of alcohol on the sexual function of women is not known. Little research has been done in this area, since the fact that women can become alcoholics has only recently become more widely accepted.

Musculoskeletal system

Acute, chronic, or subclinical myopathies can occur as a result of alcohol's deleterious effect on skeletal muscle. The exact mechanism of action is unknown, but ischemia, injury, toxicity, nutritional deficiency, impaired carbohydrate metabolism, and potassium and phosphate deficiencies have all been implicated.

Acute alcoholic myopathy is characterized by muscle pain, tenderness, and edema following excessive alcohol consumption. Symptoms subside but can recur with subsequent drinking bouts. The muscles most commonly involved are the proximal muscles of the extremities, the pelvic and shoulder girdle, and muscles of the thoracic cage.[27]

Chronic alcoholic myopathy describes a syndrome of nonpainful and nontender muscle weakness and wasting involving the same muscle groups as in acute myopathy. The onset is slow and insidious. Muscle enzymes, lactate dehydrogenase (LDH), creatine phosphokinase (CPK), and glutamic oxaloacetic transaminase (GOT), are not elevated as they are with both acute and subclinical myopathies. Subclinical alcoholic myopathy is an acute myopathy in which symptoms are absent or obscured by, for example, intoxication or withdrawal.

An increased incidence of fracture and other skeletal injuries is associated with alcoholism and occur secondarily to trauma and falls. The increased incidence of the latter is secondary to the incoordination that occurs with elevated blood alcohol levels. In addition, a syndrome of nontraumatic osteonecrosis of the hip is being recognized in excessive drinkers.[17] Fat emboli blocking end arteries have been implicated as the etiologic factor.

Integument

Skin lesions are common in alcoholic persons. Many are linked to liver disease.[33] Scratch marks may suggest abnormalities of the liver resulting in skin itchiness. Pruritus can exist as the only symptom of liver disease up to two years before cirrhosis can be diagnosed by laboratory or clinical examination.[34] Grayish skin pigmentation, diminished body hair, a purple cyanosed discoloration of the tongue, and a split in the tongue's upper surface are other stigmata of the skin and mucous membrane that can accompany liver disease. Other skin vascular changes include spider nevi and palmar erythema, a spotlike redness of the skin of the thumb and the ball of the little finger especially visible when the hand is straightened.[34]

Other skin lesions occur as a result of nutritional deficiencies, for example, glossitis secondary to folate deficiency. In addition, alcohol depresses circulating platelets, giving rise to the tendency of alcoholic patients to bruise readily.[14] The reddened, thickened skin covering the nose is commonly labeled "drinker's nose" and may be related to chronic alcohol consumption but has other causes as well, such as acne rosacea. Poor personal hygiene along with blood dyscrasias of the red and white blood cells common to alcoholic people contribute to an increased incidence of skin infections that heal poorly, such as psoriasis, seborrheic dermatitis, and "wine sores."

Hematologic system

Alcohol's adverse effect on hematopoiesis results in abnormalities of both red and white blood cells as well as platelets. Anemias, difficulty in counteracting infections, and inadequate blood clotting are clinically evident. The frequency and severity of infections of all types are increased in alcoholic persons. Multiple hematomas may be present and are a frequent indicator of an alcohol problem. Complete blood cell counts can verify the presence of anemia and/or leukopenia. Alcohol's inhibition of folate metabolism is the likely etiologic factor in these blood abnormalities.

Fetal alcohol syndrome

See Chapter 5 for a discussion of the fetal alcohol syndrome.

PSYCHOSOCIAL ASPECTS

A number of psychosocial traits are sufficiently common in alcoholic persons to merit attention. Those most frequently observed include the defense mechanisms of denial, projection, and rationalization as well as manipulation, depression and suicide, loneliness, dependency, and indicators of social deterioration. The relative predominance of any one of these in a given person is a matter of individual differences.

Defense mechanisms

The three most common defense mechanisms encountered when interviewing alcoholic people are denial, rationalization, and projection. *Denial* is frequently described as the hallmark of the alcoholic person. It is defined as the negation of reality by means of fantasy.[23] Alcoholic people use denial because they mirror society's belief that alcoholism is a shameful condition and should not occur. Additional reasons for the alcoholic person's use of denial include the need to protect a *negative self-concept,* to shield against the recognition of extreme *guilt* about behavior connected with drinking, and to maintain the false belief that the use of alcohol can be curtailed whenever desired in spite of ample evidence to the contrary.

The use of denial occurs on a continuum. On the one extreme, psychotic denial is present when no amount of reason can sway a fixed idea. Normal denial, on the opposite end, does not involve a blanket, unequivocal ignoring of reality, and rational thought can break through it. The behavior of alcoholic people falls somewhere between psychotic and normal denial, and they sway between wish and reality. When their lives are moving in a relatively manageable fashion, and the wish to drink is dominant, denial of alcoholism is extreme.[3] At this time alcoholic persons might insist that alcohol is not a problem for them and they can quit when they want to. When reality intrudes, such as after a job loss incurred as a result of frequent bouts of intoxication, denial is weak. Alcoholic persons are frequently seen in health care settings when some crisis, especially a physiologic one, has occurred in their lives. At such a time they have been referred to as being in a "sick, sad, and sorry" state and often are more receptive to intervention in their alcohol problems. They may see more clearly the effect that alcohol has on their lives. Later, when their lives are in a state of balance and denial is strong again, it is usually a less opportune time for motivating the person to change drinking habits.

Factors that simulate denial and lead to a false diagnosis if appraised inaccurately are blackouts, repression, euphoric recall, and confusion about what is occurring as alcoholism progresses.[15, 30] *Blackouts* (see Physiologic Aspects) refer to periods of amnesia caused by high blood alcohol levels. An alcoholic person seemingly denying his behavior might not, in fact, even remember it. Repression, suppression, and euphoric recall refer to selective memory of different types. *Repression* is a defense mechanism by which the alcoholic person unconsciously forgets what would be extremely anxiety producing to remember. On the other hand, an alcoholic person may consciously decide to suppress distressing or painful thoughts. *Suppression* is the conscious analog of repression and refers to the intentional exclusion of unwanted thoughts or impulses from awareness.[25] *Euphoric recall* is similar and refers to the selective remembering of pleasant events. Thus, at a party with friends, an alcoholic may spill a bloody mary on the host's white plush carpet and create other disruptions. His spouse and friends will take him to task over the episodes at a later time, whereas he will scoff and insist that he was the life of the party with his good jokes. Again, the alcoholic person is not knowingly denying the negative aspects of his behavior. Rather, for self-protection, he has "forgotten" that those things occurred and recalls only the good happenings.

Another dilemma confronting alcoholic people that superficially appears to be denial is their lack of understanding of what is happening to them because they are confused by the evidence.[30] Some alcoholics wonder how they can have problems with alcohol when they do not experience negative happenings each time they drink and do not "get drunk" each drinking occasion. In addition, alcoholic persons are likely to recall early, pleasant episodes of mild intoxication and want to reexperience them in subsequent drinking episodes. And finally, alcoholic persons may have very real difficulty in accepting alcoholism as a reality if much of their life is still in order. Frequently heard are statements such as, "I can't be an alcoholic because I haven't lost my job or my wife," or "I've never been arrested when drinking so I can't be an alcoholic."

As alcoholism becomes more problematic for the drinking person, the defense of *projection*, attributing negative interpersonal characteristics to others, is increasingly mobilized. Others are seen as guilty for any negative eventuality that occurs because of drinking. Associated with this process is the defensive maneuver of *rationalization*, whereby the alcoholic person uses perceived problems as excuses for drinking. Following are typical examples: "If you had a husband that made you stay home all the time, you'd drink too." "If your wife nagged like mine, you'd know why I need a drink to start the day off right." "Believe me, with work conditions like mine, the only way to survive is to drink." The reasons are endless. What is typical is that alcoholic persons negate all responsibility for the situation and see alcohol as the only way to cope. They also try to convince others, including nurses, that they are justified in doing as they do.

Manipulation

Alcoholic persons are often identified as being manipulators. To appraise for manipulation accurately in any one situation, and not just assume it is occurring, it is useful to keep the four characteristics of manipulative behavior in mind.[5] First, it must involve a *conflict of goal* between the manipulator and the other person. Second, the behavior must be *intentional*. Third, the behavior must be *deceptive;* one party must fully intend to "pull the wool" over the other party's eyes. Fourth, associated with this is the manipulator's feelings of *exhilaration at having put something over on the other party*. An example of manipulation is the following.

An alcoholic person about to complete a treatment program reports to the nurse to receive his daily Antabuse. The nurse's goal is to dispense the medication accurately and to have the client take it. On this particular occasion the client is planning a drinking binge and therefore does not want to take the Antabuse. He intends to deceive the nurse by pretending to take the Antabuse, keeping it in his mouth and not swallowing it. As he walks away from the nurse after doing this, he feels exhilarated at accomplishing his goal and excited about the prospective drinking bout.

Manipulation need not be a frustrating experience for the nurse if it is recognized and thwarted. The following behaviors may indicate that manipulation is occurring[4]:

1. Vying for leadership or control. The alcoholic person who is always acting superiorly exemplifies this behavior.
2. Making many demands. "My withdrawal is getting worse. I need some medication. Quick!"
3. Pressuring a person or forcing an issue. "You never pay attention to me when I tell you my concerns."
4. Violating rules, routines, procedures. Examples are the people who sneak alcohol into hospital rooms so that they will not be deprived of their drug.
5. Requesting special privileges. "My 3-year-old nephew will be in town for 2 days. May I have a pass to go see him?"
6. Playing staff and patients off; playing staff against each other. An example of the former is one patient saying to another: "I heard the head nurse say you wouldn't get any more medication because you've had enough." An example of the latter is, "The night nurse gives me extra pills so I can sleep at night, why won't you?"
7. Threatening. "I'm going to tell the doctor you refuse to give me what she orders and I'm not recovering because of it."
8. Betraying confidences. Sharing confidential group information with persons who did not participate in the group session is an example.

Confronting the alcoholic person with an awareness of the manipulative behavior can be useful in handling all four elements of the manipulative process. The goal of the confrontation is to resolve the immediate issue effectively.

Depression and suicide

Alcoholic persons often feel "down in the dumps" and "blue." Some use this as an excuse to drink; others call it an effect of drinking, and some claim both. Depression is common among alcoholic persons and may be explained, in part, by the feelings of helplessness, hopelessness, discouragement, and low self-esteem that are so prevalent in alcoholic persons. The chronic nature of alcoholism with its repeated relapses contributes to such feelings.

If a person has made any attempt to stop drinking and failed, he is likely to feel helpless and hopeless. "It's no use" and "I might as well not try" are frequently heard statements of discouragement by alcoholic persons. These feelings mount if repeated failures occur or if personal failure in some other life sphere occurs in addition. As a result, self-esteem decreases and alcoholic persons often begin to wonder what value they have as individuals if they cannot even control their drinking. They may not consider life worth living and actively contemplate and carry out suicide.

It has been estimated that the suicide rate among alcoholic persons is thirty-two times that of the general population.[26] The number of those who have considered suicide but not carried it out is still greater.

Loneliness

In the course of chronic alcoholism, those affected generally lose meaningful relationships with others and even the social skills required to form new relationships. This happens in part because their inconsistency and behavior while drunk drive others away. In addition, they are unable to communicate the reasons for their actions to others so they communicate by defensive maneuvers that serve to further separate them from others. As a result, they become unaccepted, isolated, and lonely.

It is important to understand the difference between lonesomeness, aloneness, and loneliness. Lonesomeness is a common experience that refers to the condition of being without the company of others but recognizing a wish to be with others.[24] Steps can be taken to alleviate it. Aloneness also implies being without company but by choice. It is possible to be alone without being lonesome or lonely. Loneliness, on the other hand, is not a chosen state. It can be defined as an unnoticed inability to do anything while alone.[24]

Real loneliness defies description. It is incommunicable by one who suffers it. Loneliness is characterized by paralyzing hopelessness and unutterable futility.[9] People cannot consciously endure such a painful state for very long. Consequently, loneliness is defended against and hidden.

The lonely person's self-concept is distorted. He is cut off from himself and unable to see himself as a clearly defined entity.[21] Along with this lack of self-definition go general attitudes such as worthlessness, powerlessness, and uselessness.[24] Lonely people come to feel so badly about themselves that they lose hope that they will ever care for anyone again and vice versa. They avoid their inner experience at all costs. Associated with this lack of introspection is difficulty in changing behavior patterns. So loneliness persists.

It has been said that addiction rescues from the abyss of loneliness.[22] Excessive consumption of alcohol temporarily quiets these painful feelings. The blur of intoxication is a haven for people who are lonely.

Dependency

Clinically, alcoholic persons present as dependent people. Expression of dependent behavior in adults, especially men, is negatively sanctioned in this society. It has been suggested that the conflict between dependency needs and the inability to express them leads some people to drink excessively.[10] Three possible solutions have been identified that can occur as a person attempts to resolve the conflict: open dependence, counterdependence, and alternators. A different set of observable behaviors is characteristic of each solution.

Openly dependent persons admit to dependency needs and rely heavily on others for care. The "revolving door" alcoholic person, one who seeks detoxification and treatment only to be discharged and resume drinking, endlessly repeating the cycle, is an example of an openly dependent person. The counterdependent person attempts to cover up dependency needs by acting excessively independent and powerful. This is the person who "drinks like a man" and becomes aggressive while drunk. Alternators fluctuate between openly displaying and denying dependency needs according to current life situations. Thus these persons exhibit behavior of both openly dependent and counterdependent persons.

Two characteristics also frequently seen in alcoholic persons are *impulsiveness* and *low frustration tolerance*. These behaviors are frequently described as leading people to drink. An impulsive alcoholic person is one who takes a drink almost reflexively. When asking what made him begin drinking on any particular occasion, one can expect a typical reply of "I don't know. Before I knew it, I was opening a can of beer."

Persons with a low frustration tolerance are those who get easily upset over seemingly minor occurrences. Being upset and frustrated are frequently cited as reasons to drink. Such persons have learned to deal with reality by obliterating it with alcohol rather than puzzling out distressful feelings.

Social deterioration

Two social problems encountered by a large number of alcoholic persons are economic problems and arrest and imprisonment for alcohol-related crimes. *Economic difficulties* are encountered by alcoholic persons because of the ever larger amount of money that is spent on alcohol. A continual financial drain occurs. In addition to spending a lot of money on ensuring an adequate drug supply, many alcoholic persons are fired, laid off, or quit their jobs. Thus their income may become virtually nonexistent while their spending habits may change only by purchasing a cheaper alcoholic beverage. Many alcoholics and/or their families therefore may go on welfare to make ends meet, thus increasing the social costs of alcoholism.

Employed alcoholic persons cost employers and consumers much money in terms of absenteeism and impaired work performance while on the job, including decreased efficiency and increased accidents. The effect of alcoholic employees on industry has been called "the billion dollar hangover."

In addition to financial plight, alcoholic persons may face *incarceration* for alcohol-related offenses such as driving while intoxicated (DWI) and other traffic offenses, assault, robbery (frequently to obtain money to buy alcohol), rape, and homicide. It has been estimated that approximately one half of all traffic fatalities and one third of all traffic injuries are alcohol related.[28] Information on the role of alcohol in crime is limited, but where crime is alcohol related, there are often both a drinking offender and a drinking victim. As many as 83% of offenders in prison or jail have reported alcohol involvement in their crimes, but no causal relationship between drinking problems and crime can be assumed, since prisoners seem to have more problems of all kinds than the general public.[28] However, nurses working in jails and prisons encounter a large number of alcoholic clients.

REFERENCES

1. Ansbaugh, P.: Emergency management of intoxicated patients with head injuries, Journal of Emergency Nursing 3:9, May/June, 1977.
2. Beard, J. D., and Knott, D. H.: Fluid and electrolyte balance during acute withdrawal in chronic alcoholic patients, Journal of the American Medical Association 204:133, 1968.
3. Blane, H.: The personality of the alcoholic, New York, 1968, Harper & Row, Publishers.
4. Burgess, A. W., and Lazare, A.: Psychiatric nursing in the hospital and the community, Englewood Cliffs, N.J., 1976, Prentice-Hall, Inc.
5. Bursten, B.: The manipulative personality, Archives of General Psychiatry 26:318, 1972.
6. Ettinger, P. O., et al.: Arrhythmias and the "holiday heart": alcohol associated cardiac rhythm disorders, American Heart Journal 95:55, 1978.
7. Fenster, L. F.: Alcohol and disorders of the gastrointestinal system. In Estes, N. J., and Heinemann, M. E., editors: Alcoholism, St. Louis, 1977, The C. V. Mosby Co.
8. Freund, G.: Diseases of the nervous system associated with alcoholism. In Tarter, R. E., and Sugerman, A. A., editors: Alcholism, Reading, Mass., 1976, Addison-Wesley Publishing Co., Inc.
9. Fromm-Reichmann, F.: Loneliness, Psychiatry 22:1, 1959.
10. Gorad, S. L., McCourt, W. F., and Cobb, J. C.: A communications approach to alcoholism, Quarterly Journal of Studies on Alcohol 32:651, 1971.
11. Graham, D. Y., and Davis, R. E.: Acute upper gastrointestinal hemorrhage: new observations of an old problem, American Journal of Digestive Diseases 23:76, 1978.

12. Hammond, K.: Blood ethanol, Journal of the American Medical Association **226**:63, 1974.
13. Hershon, H.: Learning to be an alcoholic, Journal of Psychosomatic Research **21**:297, 1977.
14. Hillman, R. S.: Hematological disorders of alcoholism. In Estes, N. J., and Heinemann, M. E., editors. Alcoholism, St. Louis, 1977, The C. V. Mosby Co.
15. Johnson, V.: I'll quit tomorrow, New York, 1973, Harper & Row, Publishers.
16. Kissin, B., and Begleiter, H.: The biology of alcoholism. Vol. 2, Physiology and behavior, New York, 1972, Plenum Press, Inc.
17. Leiber, C. S.: The metabolic aspects of alcoholism, Baltimore, 1977, University Park Press.
18. Lindros, K. O.: Acetaldehyde—its metabolism and role in the actions of alcohol. In Israel, Y., et al.: Research advances in alcohol and drug problems, Vol. 4, New York, 1978, Plenum Press, Inc.
19. Lovber, S. H., Dinoso, V. P., and Chey, W. Y.: Diseases of the gastrointestinal tract. In Kissin, B., and Begleiter, H., editors: Biology of alcoholism. Vol. 3, Clinical pathology, New York, 1973, Plenum Press, Inc.
20. Lyon, H. A., and Saltzman, A.: Diseases of the respiratory tract in alcoholics. In Kissin, B., and Begleiter, H., editors: Biology of alcoholism. Vol. 3, Clinical pathology, New York, 1973, Plenum Press, Inc.
21. Moustakas, C. E.: Loneliness, Englewood Cliffs, N. J., 1961, Prentice-Hall, Inc.
22. Ottenberg, D. J.: Addiction as metaphor, Alcohol Health and Research World p. 18, Fall, 1974.
23. Paredes, A.: Denial, deception, maneuvers and consistency in the behavior of alcoholics, Annals of the New York Academy of Sciences **233**:23, 1974.
24. Peplau, H.: Loneliness, American Journal of Nursing **55**:1476, 1955.
25. Peterson, M. H.: Understanding defense mechanism, American Journal of Nursing **72**:1651, 1972.
26. Seixas, F. A.: The course of alcoholism. In Estes, N. J., and Heinemann, M. E., editors: Alcoholism, St. Louis, 1977, The C. V. Mosby Co.
27. Smith, J. W.: Neurological disorders in alcoholism. In Estes, N. J., and Heinemann, M. E., editors.: Alcoholism, St. Louis, 1977, The C. V. Mosby Co.
28. United States Department of Health, Education, and Welfare: Alcohol and health, Vol. 3, Washington, D.C., 1978, U.S. Government Printing Office.
29. Van Thiel, D. H., and Lester, R.: Alcoholism: its effect on hypothalamic pituitary gonadal function, Progress in Hepatology **71**:318, 1976.
30. Wallace, J.: Alcoholism from the inside out: a phenomenological analysis. In Estes, N. J., and Heinemann, M. E., editors: Alcoholism, St. Louis, 1977, The C. V. Mosby Co.
31. Wallgren, H.: The mechanisms for actions of ethanol on the nervous system. In Ideström, C-M.: Recent advances in the study of alcoholism, Amsterdam-Oxford, 1977, Excerpta Medica.
32. Welch, C. C.: Alcoholic heart disease, Postgraduate Medicine **61**:138, 1977.
33. Whitfield, C. L., and Williams, K., editors: The patient with alcohol and other drug problems, Springfield, Ill., 1976, Whitfield and Williams.
34. Woeber, K.: The skin in diagnosis of alcoholism. In Seixas, F., Williams, K., and Eggleston, S., editors: Medical consequences of alcoholism, Annals of the New York Academy of Sciences **252**:292, 1975.
35. Wolfe, S. M., and Victor, M.: The physiological basis of the alcohol withdrawal syndrome. In Mello, N. K., and Mendelson, J. H., editors: Recent advances in studies of alcoholism, Rockville, Md., 1970, National Institute of Alcohol Abuse and Alcoholism.

CHAPTER 4

Alcohol problems in special groups
racial and ethnic groups, adolescents, multidrug abusers

Most clinical models for understanding and dealing with alcoholism have in the past been based on standards for the white, middle-aged man. Such a model is inappropriate for most of the population. This chapter provides background information about racial and ethnic groups, adolescents, and multidrug abusers with emphasis on expansion of the appraisal process for these special groups. Sensitivity to the varied experiences of these groups is essential to accurate appraisal.

RACIAL AND ETHNIC GROUPS

The United States is a multiracial society. Nurses are frequently called on to render care to different racial and ethnic groups such as black, American Indian, Hispanic, and Asian persons. However, care may be inappropriate if based only on white norms. These special groups have unique reasons for drinking, different customs and rituals, and diverse rewards gained from drinking because of their ethnic group affiliation. In appraising a person belonging to a particular ethnic group, it is important to elicit which cultural influences facilitate or inhibit the drinking response. These people may either consume alcohol according to the prescriptions of their cultural group or may look to the larger, white society for rules of drinking behavior.

It is virtually impossible to generalize about black, American Indian, Hispanic, and Asian populations, since the subgroups within each larger group are extensive. There are, for example, over 450 American Indian tribes in the United States, each with its own culture, attitudes, and religious persuasion.[45] The nurse must be wary of stereotyping members of these groups, since they are not all the same. At the same time generalization is essential to begin to heighten awareness of and sensitivity to the differences of multiracial groups from the dominant white society. The negative estimation placed on being different from the dominant group has contributed to a lowered self-concept for many members of diverse ethnic groups. Added to this is the close relationship between low self-concept and alcoholism irrespective of racial group. Although there are commonalities among members of these ethnic groups, searching for the unique aspects of each individual is an essential nursing endeavor.

The issue of poverty often overrides cultural factors. Thus persons may act in certain ways as a result of poverty rather than because of their ethnic background. Characteristics of poverty include an orientation to the present and women as heads of households, as well as feelings of hostility, fatalism, dependence, helplessness, and inferiority.

Blacks

Alcohol abuse is the major health and social problem among blacks in the United States.[22] Heavy drinking is especially prominent among poor men in urban communities and in various rural communities where bootleg liquor, taverns, and package stores are accessible.[22] Alcohol problems also occur in young blacks who have experienced childhood disruptions such as broken homes.[33,46]

Black alcoholics tend to be younger than white alcoholics, and the onset of alcoholism tends to occur earlier. Social indicators and correlates of heavy drinking and problem drinking among blacks, especially men, include poverty, truancy and failure early in school, and family instability.[23]

The habitual ingestion of alcohol by urban black men is several times higher than that for a cross section of urban men.[22] Men who can hold their liquor are held in high regard by blacks, since drinking is the norm and is not seen as a problem. Blacks also tend to use alcohol as a prestige symbol and to buy high-quality liquor. For example, although the American black population is about 11%, they buy over 30% of the Scotch sold in the United States.[37]

Blacks tend to drink excessively or not at all. Those who abstain from the consumption of alcohol do so largely for religious reasons, and since more black women than men are religious, more women are abstainers.[22]

Causative factors

Some factors in the lives of black persons lead them into a partnership with alcohol. Their position in the United States has been and still is precarious and uncertain, one that may foster frustration and a desire to escape reality. Many would rather live for the moment than defer for future gain when the prospects for change are dim. Heavy drinking increases during periods of unemployment.[40] Blacks also face poor housing and lack of upward mobility in addition to the social and psychological discrimination resulting from the fact of their being black. Thus they are in most circumstances less secure or more vulnerable to slights, slurs, or social injustices than nonblack individuals.

A well-dressed, middle-aged black woman, for example, was treated very coolly and denied permission to use the telephone at a home after her car had stalled in a predominantly white urban neighborhood. Believing that this occurred because she was black, she felt bitter and angry. Some blacks seek relief from stresses such as these in alcohol.

Black peer groups often expect one to drink and, at times, to drink heavily.[22] In addition, drinking to get "high" is a subculturally valued end in itself as well as a method for coping with painful feelings. Alcohol provides emotional release in the black community, counterbalancing the conformity and overt passivity that blacks have had to exhibit in their relationship with whites. Alcohol affords the black person a sense of personal and social power that has been unavailable in the larger society because of the alienation resulting from racism.[26]

Another factor that predisposes blacks to heavy alcohol consumption is the accessibility of liquor stores and taverns in black communities. In many inner-city neighborhoods, major supermarkets, banks, chain stores, and other services have moved out, but liquor stores and taverns remain readily available. The liquor industry is a business institution that has become interwoven into the fabric of black life.[22] For many people the tavern provides an accepted area for seeking individual recognition and for relatively uncircumscribed behavior. It is a source of company and a place that fosters mutual friendships. Blacks tend to drink in groups, since this is an accepted pattern of sociability and sharing.[22] They also tend to be heavy drinkers on weekends and holidays.

Consequences

Although alcohol often has provided blacks with a release from unpleasant realities, it has also created problems of deterioration of health, unnatural and accidental deaths, alcohol-related arrests, family disruption, and neighborhood problems.[22] Both the frequency and the magnitude of negative consequences related to alcoholism are greater for blacks than for whites. Blacks, for instance, enter treatment more often through the legal system than do whites. They have higher arrest rates because of their tendency to drink in public places and because the fact of their being black often causes them to be singled out. Alcohol-related assaults, homicides, and accidents occur more frequently among blacks than whites.[22] Personal and social problems related to heavy drinking are more severe.

It also seems that a relationship exists between alcohol withdrawal pathology and the physical environment. The more deprived the environment, the more severe the withdrawal process.[35] This may be the result of nutritional deficits and other deleterious consequences from such an environment. Since the environment of a large proportion of blacks is substandard, they are likely to suffer more intense negative physiologic consequences if they attempt to stop drinking. The added environmental stresses and risk factors increase their daily adaptive demands. Physical debilitation may be a consequence.

Physical deterioration from alcohol-related illnesses in general is greater among blacks than whites primarily because blacks tend not to seek help with physical problems until they are unable to perform their activities of daily living such as work. As long as a black person can work, he does not consider himself ill. The increased severity in the course of alcoholism and consequent symptom patterns seem to be a consequence of socioeconomic rather than racial differences largely because of the environmental demands described.[32]

Special findings

There is an increased incidence of hypertension and sickle cell anemia among the black population. Excessive alcohol use may exacerbate clinical consequences of these conditions. Hypertension, for example, is a common occurrence during withdrawal from alcohol. The high-salt, high-fat diet of blacks predisposes to the development of hypertension and exacerbates it when present. A black with high blood pressure is at extra risk for deleterious consequences during alcohol withdrawal. In addition, alcohol consumption can cause anemias because of alterations in red blood cell production and survival.[24] An alcohol-associated anemia, compounding sickle cell anemia, could severely compromise an affected individual's physiologic status. Also, painful vaso-occlusive sickle cell crises may be triggered by the physical stress of the withdrawal syndrome.

Approaches in appraisal

Language may be a factor in making an accurate appraisal of a black for an alcohol problem. Alcohol-related language used by blacks often differs significantly from that used by whites. For example, "antifreeze" refers to alcohol, a "bent number" is one who is drunk, and a "corner" refers to the last remaining drink in a bottle.[22] Since such terms are not generally understood, it is important to clarify the meanings of words the person might use. It is better to ask a meaning than to feign knowledge. Ignorance will eventually make itself known. Asking clients about use of language legitimizes their viewpoint and style, indicates concern about accurate communication, and conveys interest in them as unique individuals.

When appraising a black person for the existence of an alcohol problem, the nurse needs to look to the client for clues about the appropriateness of nonverbal behavior. Many black persons are uncomfortable with direct, sustained eye contact and regard it as "staring." On the street such eye contact indicates a confrontation. On the other hand, an upper class black person may be comfortable with sustained eye contact. In contrast, whites may interpret lack of eye contact as meaning that a person is lying or generally untrustworthy. Physical proximity or touch may not be appropriate with certain clients.

Frequently additional appraisal data can be collected from the extended family, which for many blacks is a viable, supportive system. The entire family may be involved when one member is ill or faces some other problem. The nurse must be sensitive, however, to the fact that many families are reluctant to share information about intimate matters with a stranger. The nurse must inform family members that some knowledge of the client and his activities of daily family life is essential in planning appropriate management strategies. Furthermore, the family needs to know that such information is confidential and will be used only to assist the client in his recovery from alcoholism as well as the family as it copes with that change.

Implications for prevention and treatment

To effect long-term change in the alcoholism rate among blacks, the social stresses with which they must cope, for example, racism and poverty, must be ameliorated. Changing the social environment and increasing the chances for improved living conditions and opportunities are critical prevention goals. In addition, businesses other than taverns could locate in black neighborhoods, serving to decrease the ready supply of alcohol and to eliminate a place of camaraderie for a drinking peer group. On an individual level, education about the fact that alcohol decreases rather than increases the ability of black persons to cope with the particular stresses they face may be useful.

Treatment approaches involving family support have been alluded to in the previous section. In addition, the nurse working with black alcoholic persons must be aware that they are likely to be physically debilitated and have multiple problems. Thus it may take a long time to effect recovery and return to optimum functioning. It is important to treat the other problems, for example, hypertension, along with the alcoholism. Implications for treatment also rest with broad-scale social changes focused on solutions to problems of racial and economic oppression.

American Indians and Alaskan natives

The Indian Health Service considers alcoholism a high-priority health problem that has reached epidemic proportions among American Indians and Alaskan natives. Probably no other condition adversely affects so many aspects of Indian life in the United States. The overall alcoholism death rate for the American Indian during the past few years is approximately 4.3 to 5.5 times that of all races in the United States.[45]

Prevalence

Drinking seems to be widespread, reaching its highest frequency in the 25- to 44-year age group, with men outnumbering women 3 to 1. However, not all American Indians drink; members of the Native American Church, for example, recommend abstinence.

Causative factors

The prevalence of heavy drinking among American Indians, as with blacks, is partly the result of historic and racial factors. Some tribes drank alcoholic beverages prior to the arrival of European settlers on the American continent, but the beverages were wines or beers and reserved for special, usually ceremonial and religious occasions. Hard liquor was unknown, and the Indian societies had no traditional means of coping with this product. The initial reaction to hard liquor was positive, and its effects were consonant with the spiritual experiences that were so valued by American Indians.[29]

As whites began to encroach on and undermine American Indian society and culture, the liquor trade grew and prospered. Intimately connected with the collapse of many American Indian cultures, alcohol abuse rapidly became a problem.

As early as the seventeenth century, thoughtful American Indian leaders recognized the real and potential gravity of the alcohol problem. As a result of petitions to the President as well as congressional action, the first general statutory prohibition on liquor traffic on American Indian lands was passed in 1832. It was not repealed until 1953. This was a form of prohibition that was difficult, if not impossible, to enforce. Bootleggers flourished. The illegality of drinking may have increased its appeal especially for adolescents and young adults. During this time a pattern developed of drinking until all available liquor was gone because it was less of a crime to be arrested for drunkenness than to be in actual possession of liquor. This pattern has endured. American Indians today tend to drink to get drunk and to keep drinking until the alcohol supply is exhausted.

For many American Indian problem drinkers the use of alcohol seems to be their means of dealing with anger and frustration. It could be a substitute for the powerlessness engendered by the deculturation process and the loss of many traditional tribal ways, especially when American Indians leave the reservation to find work in urban areas.[26] Many are successful in making the adjustment and lead satisfying lives. For others, however, the change of environment brings new stresses in addition to the old. Cut off from their circle of friends and relatives, a few American Indians do not successfully adapt to urban living.[42] Lack of job opportunities, boredom, inferior education, prejudice, and sometimes a language barrier precipitate heavy drinking to overcome feelings of powerlessness and lack of self-respect resulting from an inability to surmount all these barriers.[26] Many return to the reservation even more discouraged, whereas others drift into the slum section of the city where increasingly harmful drinking may be the outcome.

For the most part American Indian drinking occurs in peer or extended family groups. Alcoholic beverages, most often beer and wine, are freely shared within the group. There is strong pressure on group members both to be generous and to accept the generosity of others. These are cultural norms and apply to all material things. Intoxication is common, as described, but it is not an inevitable outcome of these episodes.

The different patterns of American Indian drinking can be partially understood in terms of historic, cultural, and social factors. Physiologic differences, especially possible differences in alcohol metabolism, are other areas of focus in attempting to clarify the patterns and effects of Indian drinking. Research reports are conflicting and cite either slower[16] or faster[17,53] alcohol metabolism among American Indians. Such possible variations require further validation.

Consequences

The adverse effects of alcoholism in the American Indian population are considerable. A majority of suicides, murders, accidental deaths, and injuries are associated with excessive drinking, as are most cases of infection, cirrhosis of the liver, and malnutrition.[42] By far the majority of arrests, fines, and imprisonments among Indians are for drinking or are the results of drinking. The associated loss of productivity and consequent abnormal social adjustments are by-products of considerable impact.

Approaches in appraisal

American Indian drinking patterns cannot be judged according to white norms for drinking behavior. Largely because of historic factors, Indians have developed a drinking pattern that is very different from that for whites. Rapid, excessive, frequent drinking is not sufficient indication to call an Indian an alcoholic. For example, members of a Northwest American Indian tribe, who rely on fishing for their livelihood, drink daily to the point of intoxication when there is no fishing to be done. But when fishing season arrives, drinking stops and is not resumed until months later when the season is over. A nurse taking a history of an intoxicated American Indian in the off-season might hastily conclude that the client was an alcoholic person. Further interactions would only be appropriate if the nurse were aware of the larger cultural context in which the drinking took place.

Also important to appraisal is the knowledge that American Indians do not readily complain of physical discomfort. In appraisal, then, the nurse should look for nonverbal clues of discomfort. Stiffening of body parts and grimacing in an intoxicated American Indian, for example, may suggest the presence of a traumatic injury.

American Indians are oriented to the present rather than the future. Whites often work without enjoyment in the present to have something in the future. American Indians, on the other hand, are more concerned that the present be enjoyed. Establishing goals based on appraisal data is best accomplished if the nurse keeps this lack of future orientation in mind and concentrates on working with the American Indian alcoholic in the present and on short-term goals.

Time orientation is different also. An American Indian may miss or be late for an appointment because he stopped to talk with someone on the way, which is viewed as a more valuable use of time. This attitude goes counter to the white norm of being highly time conscious and could be easily misinterpreted by a nurse unaware of American Indian culture.

"American Indians have strong feelings about noninterference in the lives of others."[2] The entire appraisal process, as understood by whites, could thus be jeopardized. How can the nurse determine the drinking history if such questioning is seen as rude or ill-mannered meddling? Careful explanation as to the purpose of the questioning may help allay mistrust and apprehension. Working within the American Indian's framework can make accurate appraisal possible.

Implications for treatment

Since much of American Indian drinking takes place in groups, to alter the drinking behavior it is usually essential to reestablish membership in a group, one that gives positive reinforcement for sobriety. Alcoholics Anonymous (AA), described in Chapter 10, has traditionally been unsuccessful with American Indians perhaps because of the lack of American Indian role models or a value conflict between AA and American Indian culture. Altering traditional AA tenets to fit American Indian culture more closely, as well as having groups with American Indian models, has resulted in a stronger role for AA in the Indian communities where these changes have been made.

The Native American Church is a community group that gives strong peer support for abstinence. It also offers alternatives to drinking, thus filling the void left by the removal of alcohol. It may be possible to engage the reservation Indian into this support network, but it is less available for the urban Indian. The urban environment must be assessed for the availability of alcoholism services with which an Indian could identify. Referrals can then be made.

American Indians do have considerable strengths to counteract the deleterious effects of alcohol abuse. Solid family life, religion, and a sometimes extraordinary ability to bear physical and psychologic hardships are qualities that can be mobilized to help Indians adjust to a sober life. These can be usefully employed during the treatment process to enhance the possibility of a favorable outcome.

Hispanics

Considerable differences exist among Hispanic groups in the United States in terms of language, diet, life-style, history, and country of origin. There is also considerable variation within groups because of differences in generation, education, income, and geographic location, all of which influence the drinking pattern and need to be taken into account for appraisal purposes.

Prevalence

Estimates of the rates of alcoholism based on alcohol-related physical disorders or social consequences indicate a high rate of alcoholism among Hispanics. For example, 52% of all Mexican-Americans between the ages of 30 and 60 years of age autopsied at a medical center died of alcohol-related liver disease.[14] This compares to rates ranging from 20% to 24% for white and black men and women and Hispanic women. Drunk driving arrests also indicate that the prevalence of alcohol problems in Hispanic communities is high.[13] Crime-related statistics, however, also reflect the great numbers of police usually assigned to poor Hispanic communities. It is ironic that these same communities, however, have a paucity of alcohol treatment facilities.

Causative factors

Certain cultural factors contribute to the problem of alcohol abuse among Hispanics. One important cultural attribute is the "macho" ideal of the Hispanic man, which results in sex role differences in drinking behavior. Heavy drinking is tied in with the concept of manliness and thus is an activity reserved for men. A "real" man is one who can "hold his liquor." Drinking, and especially drunkenness, is less acceptable for women.

Being macho encourages the man to believe he is master of everything within his scope of influence. Thus it is a difficult task for him to admit that he has a problem with alcohol, that he does not have control of it. As a result, it is often late in the course of alcoholism before the Hispanic man is willing to receive treatment.

The value systems of Hispanics and whites differ in a variety of ways also. The white model of "getting ahead" is not usually valued by Hispanics. Thus when there is on-the-job or for-the-job competition, the Hispanic usually loses because he does not compete yet he feels badly about losing, since loss does not fit his concept of manliness. So he may drink to cope with this conflict.

Many Hispanics live in poverty. In addition to associated disappointments and frustrations, a large number of liquor stores are readily available in poorer parts of town.

The Catholic religion predominates in Hispanic communities. Although it does not condone drunkenness, there are no sanctions against it either. Drinking, even heavy drinking, is acceptable. Confession provides an outlet that allows the church member to be penitent. In addition, many religious feasts are celebrated with drinking. Alcohol is seen as an integral part of social occasions and festivities.

The Hispanic's often frustrating experience of not being understood because of a language difference also encourages heavy drinking. An inability to speak English increases the stress and feeling of isolation that can occur when confronting the health care system. Being greeted in his native language can be a great source of relief.[25] Speaking Spanish helps in the establishment of a therapeutic relationship and makes successful assessment and treatment more likely.

Approaches in appraisal

Hispanic culture seems to provide ample emotional security and sense of belonging to its members. Great value is placed on the ability to experience emotion and to share feelings with others.[25] The family, especially, is a strong, valuable support system. Since their culture values keeping family matters private, family members usually will not provide additional appraisal data to the nurse. A dim view is taken of dissemination of such information.

Time orientation is the present. Since the concept of responsibility is based on the values just described, attending to the immediate needs of family or friends is paramount to punctuality. Thus the nurse needs to be prepared to plan for and excuse lateness in Hispanic clients.

An open, accepting attitude is crucial to working with all racial and ethnic groups. Hispanics often respond positively to this openness. Touch can be an important and effective means of demonstrating care and concern. As with blacks, it must be used with discretion and probably would not, for example, be appropriate in initial encounters with a client concerned with acting macho.

Communication with Hispanic persons needs to be diplomatic. In their culture, concern and respect for another's feelings dictate that dignity be maintained in any interaction between two individuals. Thus their manner of expression may often be elaborate and indirect, reflecting this concept of courtesy. It may take a good deal of conversation to obtain one item of data. If nurses are aware of this, they need not feel that their communication with a Hispanic is ineffectual.

Implications for prevention and treatment

It is important for the nurse to find out the amount of time the Hispanic person has been in the United States. The degree of acculturation determines values, attitudes, and knowledge of white ways.[28] Residential treatment, for example, for a recent immigrant picked up for driving while intoxicated would probably be more detrimental than therapeutic. To remove this person from others who could identify with him and place him in an alien group would be highly anxiety producing. On the other hand, a politicized Hispanic who has resided in this country for a long period of time may have much anger and bitterness to overcome before he can eradicate his alcohol problem. He may initially justify his excessive alcohol consumption by blaming it on the adversity that many minority persons face.

When a Hispanic participates in treatment, this announces publicly that there is a problem in the household. The adult male member, the one most likely to have the drinking problem, is the autocratic head of the household. No family member would go against his wishes. These strong family ties often work against a person's getting treatment for alcoholism.

The Hispanic thinks that his drinking behavior reflects poorly on the family. Since Hispanics usually rely on the family for help, they believe family members can take care of such problems. Asking for help from others may be considered a sign of weakness or personal failure; therefore it is important for the nurse to enhance and support the family's involvement in the treatment of and recovery from alcoholism.

As is true for all ethnic groups, eradication of adverse social circumstances, such as poverty and racism, is one essential component to long-term prevention and adequate treatment of alcoholism

Asian-Americans

Rates of alcoholism among Asians in general have historically been low. This seems to be due to a combination of physiologic and cultural factors. A substantial percentage of the Asian population has a biologic sensitivity to alcohol that partly consists of facial and upper body flushing, increased heart rate, decreased blood pressure, and feelings of nausea. These aversive symptoms outweigh the pleasant effects of alcohol so that individuals with this sensitivity are protected from becoming alcoholic.[54]

In addition to this physiologic damper to heavy drinking, Asian cultural attitudes toward intoxication are negative and alcoholism is stigmatized.[4] As a result, their drinking patterns in general are more moderate and drinking to the point of drunkenness is uncommon.

Special findings

The exact mechanism for the flushing phenomenon just noted is unknown. Flushing seems to be dose related—the more alcohol consumed, the greater the flushing. Besides the symptoms just described, it is often also accompanied by subjective symptoms of discomfort such as dizziness, pounding in the head, muscle weakness, and tingling sensations. There is speculation that the flushing may be due to racial differences in acetaldehyde levels, with Asians having higher concentrations, or variations, in autonomic reactivity.* Chinese people have been shown to absorb alcohol more quickly than whites.[54] Both Japanese and Chinese persons seem to metabolize alcohol at a significantly higher rate than Europeans, perhaps as a result of an established variant of the liver enzyme alcohol dehydrogenase.[38] Anatomic variation has been implicated in this ethnic difference in alcohol metabolic rate.[20] Asians have longer intestines and the highest relative sitting height of any group of humans. This should result in a proportionately larger liver. Flushing, then, may be related to accelerated metabolism.

The traditionally moderate drinking pattern of Asians appears to be changing. Alcoholism is on the rise in Japan, for example. It would appear that as Japanese culture becomes more exposed to that of the West, some of the negative sanctions against drinking are lost as new, heavier drinking patterns are adopted.

Asian-Americans in general prefer personal rather than professional approaches for amelioration of health problems, including alcoholism. Help would be sought in the community, from family members and friends, rather than in health care institutions from professionals.[4] For example, an Asian-American may seek a consultation with an herb doctor rather than a physician. Individual nurses working in the community may become sufficiently trusted so that an Asian-American becomes comfortable in sharing drinking-related concerns with them.

As an example, a middle-aged Chinese-American woman had been having abdominal pain for approximately 2 weeks when she decided to allow her daughter to have a friend, a nurse, come to see her. The appraisal took place in the client's home over tea. (It was crucial to make this woman feel at ease. Drinking tea with her helped immensely.) The woman spoke no English and her daughter interpreted. The daughter stated that her mother had been drinking a pint of sake daily for the past four years. Lately she had increased her daily amount to alleviate some of the pain she was experiencing. When examined by the nurse, she had alcohol on her breath. It was 11 AM on a Sunday morning. In addition to increasing her drinking, the woman had tried a variety of home remedies in attempts to relieve the pain, none of which had worked. The pain was becoming more intense; she was having difficulty eating and could not afford to lose weight.

After obtaining this information through careful questioning, the nurse examined the woman's abdomen. In doing so, it was important to protect her modesty carefully, continue to talk with her, and keep her at ease. The right upper quadrant of her abdomen was exquisitely tender to light palpation. The nurse encouraged her to go to

---

*References 15, 31, 49, 50, 54.

a physician for a follow-up examination. The woman was hesitant because of her discomfort about being examined by a man. To help her feel more at ease, a Chinese woman physician was chosen and her daughter accompanied her. After further tests a duodenal ulcer was diagnosed. The following week she had a surgical repair of the lesion. When the relationship between this physical condition and her excessive drinking was explained to her, this woman was eager to get help in changing her alcohol consumption pattern. She was referred to the Asian Community Clinic for outpatient counseling. Two years later she is sober and healthy.

Success in referring this woman was at least partly the result of the nurse's responsiveness to her as an individual influenced by specific cultural beliefs. The nurse's willingness to go to the home, to drink tea, and to inquire about the use of home remedies put the patient at ease and allowed her to trust the nurse and to follow up on her suggestions.

Approaches in appraisal

The appraisal process is influenced by the Asian-American emphasis on social and interpersonal values. The foremost of these is smooth interpersonal relationships manifested by pleasant, polite, agreeable behavior and a courteous respect for the ways and wishes of others. In addition, Asian-Americans tend to take problems to family or friends initially. Because of these two factors, it is often difficult for an Asian-American person to acknowledge true feelings and to take an active part in the appraisal interview. He needs to feel that he can trust the nurse first, then with time he will open up and share personal thoughts and feelings.

Asking the client about quantity of alcohol consumed in a specified period of time might elicit a response in "teacupsful" because alcohol is consumed from teacups. For conversion purposes a teacupful is approximately 90 ml. In a recent health needs assessment in the Seattle Asian-American community, some persons reported consuming 10 teacupfuls of liquor daily. Health professionals in the area were surprised by the frequency with which alcohol consumption was reported, attesting to what seems to be a trend toward increased, and often problematic, alcohol consumption among Asian-Americans.

Implications for prevention and treatment

Because of the Asian-American reliance on the family and traditional health care practitioners, such as herb doctors, trust is only shared with professional persons, including nurses, when they demonstrate genuine interest in the well-being of their Asian clients. In terms of case finding, it is crucial that nurses be out in the community so that they can observe disruptive drinking patterns because they will most likely not be sought out until physical health has deteriorated. Likewise, if the nurse is accessible to the community, family members might seek her out on an informal basis to talk about alcoholism.

ADOLESCENTS

During the past several decades there has been a growing concern in the United States about both alcohol and other drug use among young people. Much of the attention in the 1960s focused on youngsters from middle class America who were using illicit substances such as LSD and marijuana. The 1970s saw a return to alcohol as the preferred drug of youth together with the retention of other drugs, especially marijuana.

Experimentation with alcohol seems to be a normal part of growing up for most adolescents in this society. Although all states have legal drinking ages, varying from 18 to 21 years, these laws have not deterred the majority of youths from drinking alcohol. Most young people have at least tried alcohol by the time they leave high school.[43] By the late 1970s the use of alcohol by youth had become so pervasive and socially accepted or tolerated that its potential destructiveness was sometimes overlooked.

Trends

In general, the number of adolescents who have used alcohol, usually meaning having one's own drink rather than sipping from another person's drink, at least once during the prior year has increased significantly over the last thirty years. Prior to World War II barely 25% of adolescents reported drinking, by the end of the war the number increased to over 33%, the figure jumped to 60% by the mid-1950s, to almost 70% by the mid-1960s and to between 80% and 90% by the mid-1970s.[36]

In an era of changing sex roles, the most significant recent change in patterns of drinking has been the great increase in drinking by girls. Differences in drinking rates between the sexes have all but disappeared.[9] Generally speaking, boys tend to prefer to drink beer and whiskey, whereas girls show some predilection for wine.[6]

Multidrug use is a trend among teenagers in the 1970s. Youth not only have alcohol but the drugs of the 1960s as well. Combining alcohol and nicotine, alcohol and marijuana, and alcohol alterated with uppers such as amphetamines or cocaine are examples of multidrug use.

Teenagers typically are introduced to alcohol by their families in their own homes. Currently their first drinking experience usually occurs around 12 years of age compared with the 1940s and 1950s when it happened at 13 to 14 years.[9] The amount and frequency of drinking increases with age,[30] and over 6% of high school seniors report daily alcohol use.[1]

Adolescents exposed to parents, peers, and religious systems that approve of drinking are more likely to be drinkers themselves. Teenage abstainers are less exposed to drinking cultures and are more likely to have nondrinking parents and peers and to perceive their church or religion as disapproving of drinking.[21]

Problem drinkers

Most adolescents use alcohol in nondestructive ways, drinking temperately and infrequently. At the same time there is an alarming number of teenagers with drinking problems, and this number appears to be growing.

Although there is no single accepted definition of adolescent problem drinking, it generally encompasses behaviors ranging from frequent intoxication to interpersonal and school-related complications. In addition, teenage drinkers who have increased episodes of intoxication have more trouble with the law as a result of driving while intoxicated, being found in possession of alcohol, and involvement in alcohol-related automobile accidents. In a recent national survey of students in grades 7 through 12, drinking and problem drinking was examined. It was found that 79% of the boys and 70% of the girls were drinkers. Problem drinking was defined either as drunkenness at least six times in the past year or the presence of negative consequences from drinking two or more times in at least three of five specified situations in the past year or both. Students acknowledged the following negative consequences resulting from drinking: (1) getting into trouble with teachers or a principal, (2) getting into difficulties with friends, (3) driving when having had a "good bit" to drink, (4) being criticized by someone the student was dating, and (5) getting into trouble with the police. By this definition nearly 19% of the students were problem drinkers, 23% of the boys and 15% of the girls. Problem drinking increased with age, from 5% of seventh grade boys to nearly 40% of twelfth grade boys and from 4.4% of seventh grade girls to 21% of twelfth grade girls.[11]

Figures on problem drinking may be low, since surveys are conducted on young people in school. Students who are having difficulty with alcohol are likely to be absent because of hangovers or drunkenness when the surveys are taken. School dropouts and institutionalized delinquents are not included in these surveys, and there is some evidence that drinking among dropouts is higher than for students who remain in school.[27]

The question of how accurately surveys about use of illegal substances are completed by teenagers is difficult to answer. It can be speculated that some youth, possibly those having the most difficulty with alcohol, may provide inaccurate data, making reliable figures difficult to obtain.

Adolescent problem drinking does not tend to be an isolated behavior; rather it has been found to be a part of a general adaptation to self, others, and circumstances. In the national study mentioned above consisting of data from adolescents in grades 7 through 12, problem drinkers showed a pattern of greater susceptibility to problem behavior than nonproblem drinkers. Three systems of psychosocial variables, personality, perceived environment, and behavior, were assessed in regard to susceptibility to problem drinking. In the personality systems, problem drinkers valued independence more and had lower expectations for academic achievement. They were more tolerant of transgression, less religious, and emphasized the positive functions of drinking. In the perceived environment system, problem drinkers' susceptibility to problem behavior was manifested by loosened ties with parents and a greater orientation toward their peers. In the behavior system the problem drinkers' susceptibility to problem behavior was revealed by less involvement in or commitment to conventional activities such as church and school work and a greater involvement with other drugs such as marijuana and activities such as lying, stealing, and aggression.[11]

Children of alcoholic parents are considered to be an especially high-risk group in terms of developing problem drinking. These young people are more likely than their peers to experience alcohol-related problems both during adolescence and later in life.[6]

Alcoholism

Anecdotal reports in the 1970s indicated an increase in the number of teenagers entering detoxification facilities and attending Alcoholics Anonymous. Determining the number of adolescents actually affected by alcoholism is complicated, as is adolescent problem drinking, by lack of a definition of adolescent alcoholism. An adult alcoholic is characterized as a person whose normal functioning has been disrupted by alcohol. Adolescents have not achieved a stable mode of functioning and so, with the exception of school activities, it is less clear as to where alcohol presents a disruptive influence. In regard to the physiologic aspects of alcoholism, many of these indicators only manifest themselves after long years of alcohol abuse. On this basis, some argue that adolescents cannot be regarded as alcoholic.[41] At the same time some adolescents have been treated for symptoms of alcohol withdrawal, indicative of physiologic dependence and therefore of alcoholism. There is some evidence that youth may be affected more quickly by alcohol than adults because of differences in body weight and the more critical nutritional needs of adolescents during body growth and organ development.[3]

Given the current lack of clarity regarding adolescent alcoholism, labeling an adolescent as alcoholic may be inaccurate as well as damaging to the individual's self-image. Since youth frequently experiment with alcohol, it is essential to determine if the young person's excessive involvement with alcohol is transient and only a part of "growing up" or if, indeed, it indicates a serious problem with alcohol.

Reasons for drinking

Teenagers give a variety of reasons for using alcohol. They may be curious about its taste and effects, or they may wish to participate in a widespread social custom. They live in a heavily drinking society where the majority of adults drink. Some teenagers think that drinking gives them an added dimension of maturity and view alcohol use as a rite of passage to adulthood.

Teenagers may use alcohol in response to peer pressure and to ensure their popularity within the group. The pressure from peers to drink seems to play a larger role among older adolescents. Younger adolescents are not usually required to drink even if their peer group does, and the nondrinker may be more highly regarded than the drinker. As adolescents reach their upper teens, those who deviate from the norm of drinking may be ridiculed by their peers.[6]

Drinking to get drunk or to deal with crisis, depression, or rejection are reasons more likely to be given by young problem drinkers. More important than the initial impetus to drink is the effect that continued drinking has on the adolescent and the ease with which alcohol can be adopted as an individual's chief coping mechanism.

There are no complete answers concerning why teenagers drink. In addition to the reasons cited, adolescent drinking practices often closely resemble those of their parents and, as such, are not typically an expression of rebellion and hostility toward adult authority. In this vein, teenage drinking practices can be viewed as an imitation of adult drinking patterns as perceived by the teenager. In sum, adolescents do not invent ideas of drinking or abstinence; rather they learn from their observations of adult behavior.

Consequences

Typically adults view drinking by teenagers with alarm and apprehension. What are reasons for this concern, especially as regards the consequences of teenage drinking?

Young people are naive drinkers—they lack experience with the drug alcohol. They tend to drink less frequently and to drink less on most occasions than adults. Most teenagers therefore have a low tolerance to alcohol, and they are likely to experience considerable impairment with small doses. As stated previously, physiologic symptoms consequent to the development of tolerance to alcohol usually take long periods to appear. Adolescents are less likely to experience these symptoms than adults. However, teenage drinkers do appear in health care facilities, most often as a result of overdosing on alcohol. Frequently, for example, after a major rock concert it is possible to find a number of youthful concert attenders in emergency rooms being assessed and treated for acute alcohol and other drug intoxication.

Most have been brought to the emergency room by police. Their presence may represent a single incident of heavy drinking or may be one of a long series of intoxicated episodes. Such teenagers require emergency treatment to ensure safe recovery from the acute state of intoxication, and sometimes coma, and require assessment as to the possible need for additional longer term treatment.

The phenomenon of low tolerance to and increased impairment with small doses of alcohol also inevitably creates problems with driving a car and the operation of all types of machinery for young drinkers. Youthful drivers, in general, are especially at high risk for driving problems with a peak incidence of accidents in the 18- to 19-year age range.[48] Individuals under 25 years of age are involved in almost one half of all fatal highway accidents,[34] and 60% of fatal drunk driving accidents involve teenage drivers.[36]

Another prime reason for concern about teenage alcohol use relates to the way alcohol may interfere with accomplishing the developmental tasks of adolescence. Adolescence is the period of life when young people need to prepare to cope on their own, to form intimate heterosexual relationships, and to choose some means of making a living. It is a time of many choices requiring the use of intellectual and psychological skills. Reliance on alcohol can interfere with achievement of these tasks during this critical period. When young people use alcohol to solve problems, they deprive themselves of the opportunity to learn more constructive ways of dealing with life. Frequent interference with psychologic and social maturation processes can leave the adolescent without the emotional capacity to deal with adult life. A readily available escape from this situation is to develop an even greater reliance on alcohol.

Approaches in appraisal

Teenagers rarely admit openly and spontaneously to being concerned about their alcohol or drug abuse. More often they come to the attention of health care workers because of court referrals, concerned parents, teachers, or school counselors. At the same time most teenagers have not been drinking long enough to develop physical stigmata of alcoholism. For these reasons it is essential during appraisal for the nurse to be alert to recent *behavioral* changes indicative of alcohol abuse. Following is a listing of such clues*:

Drop-off in school grades
Truancy
Disinterest in sports or hobbies to which teenager previously devoted much time

*Modified with permission by Patient Care magazine. Copyright © 1975, Patient Care Publications Inc., Darien, Conn. All rights reserved.

Changes in personal habits such as decreased interest in dress, shaving, hair, bathing

Nervousness or depression, specifically a sense of impending doom

Phobias of sudden onset that follow the "blackout" experience

Indications of suicidal tendencies—frequent expressions of feeling restless, hopeless, a failure, a nobody with nothing to do

Empty liquor bottles hidden in teenager's room

Drinking during the day, at school, or elsewhere

Withdrawal from family, friends, and classmates

Changes in social life; the desire to drink alone may cause attendance at fewer parties

Teenager's own concern that his/her drinking is different from that of friends

On appraisal of a teenager with a history of long-term alcohol abuse, the following symptoms may be elicited*:

Flushed or pallid face

Tachycardia

Hypertension

Slight tremors

Reddened, atrophic, or coated tongue

Hepatomegaly and/or hepatic tenderness

Bruises on shins and other body parts from falling or bumping into things

Alcohol on breath, or even more likely, cover-up fresheners on the breath

Verbal expression by teenagers of a psychological need for the mind-altering qualities of alcohol

Establishing oneself as trustworthy and knowledgeable is of special importance when appraising adolescent alcohol abusers. The young person needs to feel safe in confiding in the nurse and to perceive her concern for him. In establishing trust, the nurse should be herself and not use youth culture language unless thoroughly conversant with it—otherwise she is likely to come across as a phony.

Encouraging the adolescent to express his point of view regarding reasons for needing health care is useful. His ideas may differ from the opinion of parents or whoever brought him for help. Seeking and building on the adolescent's point of view, where possible, conveys an interest in helping him maintain his autonomy, a factor of considerable concern to most teenagers.

Exploring what is happening at home by including parents, siblings, or both in the appraisal interview helps to assess the teenager's behavior. Sometimes the teenager drinks excessively in response to a crisis in the family unit

---

*Modified with permission by Patient Care Magazine. Copyright © 1975, Patient Care Publications, Inc., Darien, Conn. All rights reserved.

such as divorce, physical or mental abuse, or parental alcoholism. When one or both parents are alcoholic, alcohol and other drugs are often readily available at home. Most teenagers will also need time to be interviewed individually as well as with family members and will need assurance as to the confidentiality of the interview.

Direct questioning about alcohol and drug use needs to be done slowly and initiated after the appraisal interview is well underway. Questions appropriate to teenagers, including their involvement in social and school activities and friendships with peers, are most likely to lead to informative answers. When the nurse is able to discover how the young person relaxes or spends leisure time, she may simultaneously learn about alcohol and drug use. Exploring the usual life-style of the adolescent and if or how that has changed may be revealing. For example, a high school boy who had been an outstanding football player during his sophomore and junior years ceased his sports activity when, as a senior, he began using alcohol daily. Another example is a teenager who formerly was involved with a number of peers in constructive activities, including drama productions, who now spends considerable time consuming alcohol with one or two drinking buddies.

Although many adolescents deny their involvement with alcohol, others exaggerate alcohol intake. A youthful drinker may brag about drinking half a case of beer (when in actuality he is drunk on three beers) because of a need to impress others with his ability to handle great quantities of alcohol. Sensitivity to either extreme increases the likelihood of the nurse's obtaining accurate data.

During the appraisal interview the adolescent may question the nurse about her involvement with alcohol and other drugs. It is best to be brief, honest, and factual in response to such direct questions. Young people are quick to notice and point out inconsistencies or hypocrisies on the part of adults. If this happens, responding thoughtfully and nondefensively to the adolescent's observations can provide a model of behavior for the adolescent to emulate.

Finally, during assessment it is important for the nurse to determine the chronology of symptoms. This can sometimes be accomplished in the context of determining the teenager's reasons for drinking. If, for example, excessive drinking begins following a crisis event in the young person's life, such as an unresolved grief reaction, mental health assistance may be needed along with learning to moderate or discontinue alcohol intake.

Prevention

To halt the increase in the numbers of young people with alcohol problems, greater efforts in prevention must be made. Massive educational programs responsive to the needs of youth need to be launched.

The schools are a logical place to provide prevention efforts because they reach more youth than any other single institution. It is necessary for schools to introduce content about alcohol at the earliest grade level and to build on this knowledge throughout the basic educational curriculum to have the greatest positive effect on young people's values and behavior patterns. Teachers and other adults who serve as role models need thorough education about alcohol also to deal effectively with youth on this subject. It is not enough, however, for educational programs simply to provide clear, realistic, and accurate information about alcohol. Decision-making skills and a healthy attitude about oneself are additional requisites to promote responsible behavior among youth concerning alcohol use or nonuse.

The family is also an extremely potent agent for influencing the decisions young people make about alcohol. Home atmospheres that are permissive about heavy drinking often promote the excessive use of alcohol by youth. Parents need to make certain that they are setting a good example for their children in their own drinking patterns such as by moderating its use. Many parents will need opportunities within their communities to discuss and clarify their own attitudes about alcohol before they can convincingly guide their children in this crucial area.

Peer pressure, often instrumental in influencing youth to drink, can also be used to curb drinking. Older students, who are identified as leaders and who have responsible attitudes and positive behaviors toward drinking, can serve as role models for younger students. It may be easier for some youth to identify with mature persons in their own age group than with adults. Peer-centered prevention programs have been initiated recently in several settings, and their long-term effectiveness has yet to be evaluated.[51]

Another area for prevention of alcohol problems among youth involves the media. Advertisements are used to glamorize alcohol, depicting it as an immense social asset. Young people are impressionable and easily persuaded, and mass media need to be used to communicate alcohol-problem prevention messages. Counteradvertising on radio, television, and in the press are likely to achieve a greater effectiveness when combined with follow-up such as discussion groups and community involvement.[44]

Treatment

Only in recent years has alcoholism in youth been recognized, and treatment efforts geared directly toward meeting the needs of this population are still largely in developmental stages. In most alcoholism treatment programs young clients receive the same treatment as adult clients, in some a youth component has been added, and there are a few programs solely for teenage alcohol abusers.

Conventional ways of dealing with adult alcoholic people may not work with youth. Young alcohol abusers need recovery programs that are staffed with experts in adolescent psychology who have skills in dealing with personality disturbances beyond alcohol problems. Many young people exhibit a pattern of multidrug use and require a comprehensive program of accelerated treatment not available in most existing adult-oriented programs.

Within treatment programs adolescents need ample education about alcohol and alcoholism and opportunities to explore and try out alternate ways of adjusting to life without alcohol use. Although lifelong abstinent goals are often appropriate and acceptable to adult alcoholics, adolescents may experience more overall success in a program that stresses moderation in alcohol intake.

Ongoing involvement in academic studies needs to be provided for youth who have not completed high school, and opportunities to develop vocational skills need to be made available to older adolescents who have completed basic education. Individual and group counseling and family involvement must also be stressed in programs for youth. Consultation with teachers, guidance counselors, psychologists, and school nurses is necessary to provide an orderly transition between the treatment agency and the environment to which the young person will return.

Adolescents seek adult roles, and the behavior of treatment personnel needs to exemplify maturity in all matters, but especially in regard to alcohol and other drug use. It is especially important for adults working with adolescents to be conscious of their actions, far more than their words, because by and large what adults do, youth will do.

MULTIDRUG ABUSERS

Multidrug abusers are persons who abuse more than one drug concomitantly. This phenomenon is increasing and seems to be becoming the drug consumptive pattern of choice for persons who use drugs.[18] Consumption of mood-altering drugs follows numerous patterns. Some of the heaviest users of illegal drugs are also heavy alcohol users.[5,19,39,47] The combination of drugs with alcohol is the most frequent cause of drug-related medical incidents such as overdose, death, and hospital admissions.[18]

Multidrug abuse does not exclusively indicate simultaneous drug abuse. Rather, a person's entire life might revolve around consumption of various drugs. For example, some individuals consume "uppers" to get going in the morning, alcohol at noon for temporary sedation, and prescription or over-the-counter sleeping tablets on retiring for the night. Such a person is classed as a multidrug abuser because of the consumption of many drugs.

Uniqueness

Multidrug abusers have been divided into two dichotomous categories: self-medicators versus recreational and street-wise versus nonstreet-wise users.[7,10] Since it is common for persons to shift their primary pattern of drug consumption, a person may fit into each of these categories over a period of multidrug abuse.

Self-medicators are described as distressed persons who attempt to cope with their problems through the use of drugs. They use them regularly, space out the consumption, and usually take them solitarily. These persons, often women and elderly, believe that they need the drugs to function effectively. Frequently they continue to take drugs to alleviate the discomfort that may result from drug deprivation.[10]

Recreational users, on the other hand, take drugs with other people in large amounts and sporadically in binges. They use them to get "high" and it has been suggested that they may be coping with a lack of pleasurable stimuli in their lives.[10] This illustrates that social as well as chemical factors reinforce and thus perpetuate recreational drug use.

An individual who can maintain drug usage through reliance on other than socially sanctioned means, through dealers and pushers, for example, is a street-wise drug abuser. These persons also tend to dress unconventionally, use street lingo, reside in a geographic area known as a youth drug subculture, engage in criminal activity to support themselves and their drug habit, and as a result, often get arrested.[7]

Nonstreet-wise, or straight, drug abusers, on the other hand, are older and began using drugs later in life. They have fewer arrests, a better employment history, and generally are better educated and less deviant than street-wise persons.[7] They usually obtain their drugs by means of legal and illegal prescriptions and as a result, suffer less of the deleterious consequences of drug abuse.

Classification of multidrug abusers can also occur by means of describing the pattern of multidrug use with respect to primary and secondary drugs. Such patterns originate mainly from the various motivations for abuse of particular drugs.[12] Thus alcohol may be used with secondary drugs such as the sedatives that potentiate its effects or the amphetamines that antagonize its effects. On the other hand, alcohol may be the secondary drug. Many drug addicts also drink heavily. A growing number of persons on a regimen of methadone maintenance, for example, become dependent on alcohol.[12]

Consequences

Consequences of multidrug abuse are related to the abuser's life-style as well as to the interaction of the drugs abused. Drugs can either potentiate or negate each other and have additive or synergistic effects. The casual life-style of multidrug abusers often leads to poor nutrition and, as a result, frequent infections. Intravenous or subcutaneous administration of drugs also leads to frequent infection as well as abscesses and hepatitis. Parenteral routes of administration are often tried by many multidrug abusers.

Approaches in appraisal

Changes in mood, emotions, and cycles of sleep and wakefulness may offer some clue in clients suspected of multidrug abuse.[12] Evidence of withdrawal symptoms, concomitant diseases such as hepatitis and cardiac arrhythmias, or presence of complications such as cutaneous manifestations and evidence of cross tolerance, are often extremely useful in appraising multidrug abuse problems in clients.[12]

It is often difficult to appraise the health status of multidrug abusers because of conflicting or exaggerated signs and symptoms. The combination of sedative hypnotics and alcohol, for example, may produce a coma in a person that greatly exceeds what would be expected based on blood alcohol level. The depressant effect of alcohol combined with the stimulant effect of amphetamines presents a confusing clinical picture. *It therefore is essential for the nurse, when inquiring about drug use patterns, not to assume that a person uses only one drug and stop the questioning there.* It is necessary to ask what other drugs the client uses to allow him an opportunity to continue to describe his drug use. If a client claims use of only one drug and yet the symptom picture implicates more, the nurse needs to inquire about other drug use, frankly pointing out to the client the inconsistency between history and presenting symptoms.

Communication is easier with street-wise persons, since they tend to be more open to admitting problems than straight individuals.[7] Even though the street-wise person converses readily, the nurse must be especially cautious in evaluating the content of the client's remarks and look for facts on which to appraise his condition accurately. Multidrug abusers are exceedingly adept at symptom description and will often exaggerate physical discomfort to be medicated further, especially if they are experiencing drug withdrawal. It is difficult for the nurse not to respond and to comfort them. However, objectivity must be maintained. It is important to establish a trusting relationship with these clients. In most cases, if a nurse approaches such a person with caution and kindness, he will respond in a trusting manner.[10]

The nurse's focus during the appraisal process should not be on drug abuse as the primary symptom. Such an approach assumes similarity of many drug behaviors and, as a result, ignores some profound individual differences. The straight self-medicator, for example, acknowledges more depressive affect than the street-wise, recreational user.[7] The drugs they abuse may be the same, yet their symptom pattern is different.

The interaction of the individual's personality, the desired or anticipated effects of the drugs, the person's mood when the drugs are taken, which drugs are used, and the social situation all determine drug effects.[52] Reactions to drugs taken at different times but by the same individual can vary considerably. In appraising a drug abuser for withdrawal symptoms and/or adverse reactions, the nurse can ask the person how these have been experienced before. This information may serve as a guideline but will not dictate the reactions experienced with this episode.

Implications for prevention and treatment

Prior to discussing treatment for multidrug abusers, it is prudent to mention a pattern of multidrug abuse that can be prevented. That pattern is the accidental combination of drugs in low doses which, when taken in combination, may have deleterious consequences. Alcohol, for example, when combined with other depressant drugs either prescribed or purchased over the counter, may cause coma or even death in a unsuspecting individual even when all the drugs are taken in moderation. In addition to combined drug effects, alcohol can also interfere with the absorption or metabolism of various therapeutic agents, for example, antibiotics, rendering standard doses of such medication ineffective. Clients must be informed that it is good health practice to drink nothing while taking medication. (See Chapter 6, Table 4.)

A nurse's encounter with drug abusers will often be at a time when, because of physical discomfort, their defenses are down and they are vulnerable. This is often a good time to encourage them to get help with their drug abuse problem. The best approach is firmness, not confrontation. If the nurse encroaches too closely on the client's power to make decisions, he may tighten his defenses and shut the nurse out entirely.

As a group, multidrug abusers are resistant to known treatment modalities. Treatment should be highly individualized and aimed at correcting difficulties in managing activities and demands of daily living as well as supplementing available resources. Problems in these areas can be diagnosed from information gained by careful nursing appraisal.

REFERENCES

1. The alcoholism report. **6:**6, Oct. 13, 1978, J SL Reports, 1120 National Press Bldg., Washington, D.C.
2. Baker, J.: Alcoholism and the American Indian. In Estes, N.J., and Heinemann, M. E., editors: Alcoholism, development, consequences and interventions, St. Louis, 1977, The C. V. Mosby Co.
3. Bennett, J. A., et al.: Drug spotlight: Who will help teenage alcohol abusers? Patient Care **16:**88-89; 91; 94-97; 101; 103; Sept. 15, 1975.
4. Bickerton, Y. J., and Sanders, R. V.: Ethnic preferences in alcoholism treatment: the case of Hawaii, Annals of the New York Academy of Sciences **273:**653, 1976.
5. Blum, R. H.: Drugs and students, San Francisco, 1969, Jossey-Bass, Inc., Publishers.
6. Bosma, W. G. A.: Alcoholism and teenagers, Maryland State Medical Journal **24:**62, June, 1975.
7. Carlin, A. S., and Strauss, F. F.: Descriptive and functional classifications of drug abusers, Journal of Consulting Psychology **45:**222, 1977.
8. Cartwright, A. K. J., and Shaw, S. J.: Trends in the epidemiology of alcoholism, Psychological Medicine **8:**1, Feb. 1978.

9. Demone, H. W., and Wechsler, H.: Changing drinking patterns of adolescents since the 1960s. In Greenblatt, N., and Schuckit, M. A., editors: Alcoholism problems in women and children, New York, 1976, Grune & Stratton, Inc.
10. Detzer, E., Muller, B., and Carlin, A. S.: Identifying and treating the drug misusing patient, American Family Physician **16**:181, Sept., 1977.
11. Donovan, J. E., and Jessor, R.: Adolescent problem drinking, Journal of Studies on Alcohol **39**:1506, 1978.
12. Dutta, S. N., and Kaufman, E.: Multiple drug abuse. In Pradham, S. N., and Dutta, S. N., editors: Drug abuse, St. Louis, 1977, The C. V. Mosby Co.
13. East Los Angeles Health Task Force: East Los Angeles health supplemental report: a follow-up report on the health problems and priorities in East Los Angeles, Los Angeles, June, 1972.
14. Edmanson, H. A.: Mexican-American alcoholism and deaths at LAC-USC Medical Center, Testimony before the Subcommittee on Alcoholism of the California State Health and Welfare Committee, Los Angeles, Feb. 7, 1975.
15. Ewing, J. A., Rouse, B. A., and Pellizzari, E. D.: Alcohol sensitivity and ethnic background, American Journal of Psychiatry **131**:206, 1974.
16. Everett, M. W., Waddell, J. O., and Dwight, B. H.: Cross-cultural approaches to the study of alcohol, The Hague, 1976, Morton Publishers.
17. Farris, J. J., and Jones, B. M.: Ethanol metabolism in male American Indians and whites, Alcoholism: Clinical and Experimental Research **2**:83, 1978.
18. Glatt, M. M.: Drug dependence, Baltimore, 1977, University Park Press.
19. Goode, E.: Drugs in American society, New York, 1972, Alfred A. Knopf, Inc.
20. Hanna, J. M.: Metabolic responses of Chinese, Japanese and Europeans to alcohol, Alcoholism: Clinical and Experimental Research **2**:89, 1978.
21. Harford, T. C.: Teenage alcohol use, Postgraduate Medicine **60**:73, July, 1976.
22. Harper, F. D., editor: Alcohol abuse and black America, Alexandria, Va., 1976, Douglass Publishers, Inc.
23. Harper, F. D.: Alcohol and blacks: state of the periodical literature. Unpublished paper, Howard University, Washington, D.C., 1974.
24. Hillman, R. S.: Hematological disorders of alcoholism. In Estes, N.J., and Heinemann, M. E., editors: Alcoholism, development, consequences and interventions, St. Louis, 1977, The C. V. Mosby Co.
25. Maccoby, M.: On Mexican national character. In Wagner, N. N., and Haug, M. J., editors: Chicanos, St. Louis, 1971, The C. V. Mosby Co.
26. Mohatt, G.: The sacred water: the quest for personal power through drinking among the Teton Sioux. In McClelland, D. C., et al., editors: The drinking man, New York, 1972, The Free Press.
27. Nelson, D. O.: A comparison of drinking and understanding of alcohol and alcoholism between students in selected high schools in Utah and in the Utah State Industrial School, Journal on Alcohol Education **13**:17, 1968.
28. Paine, H. J.: Attitudes and patterns of alcohol use among Mexican Americans: implications for service delivery, Journal of Studies on Alcohol **38**:544, 1977.
29. Plog, S. C., and Edgerton, R. B.: Changing perspectives in mental illness, New York, 1969, Holt, Rinehart & Winston, Inc.
30. Rachal, J. V., et al.: A national study of adolescent drinking behavior, attitudes and correlates, The Research Triangle Institute for The National Institute on Alcohol Abuse and Alcoholism, Contract No. HSM 42-73-80, prepared for the U.S. Department of Health, Education, and Welfare, April, 1975.
31. Reed, T. E., et al.: Alcohol and acetaldehyde metabolism in Caucasians, Chinese and Amerinds, Canadian Medical Association Journal **115**:851, 1976.
32. Rimmer, J., Pitts, F. N., Reich, T., and Winokur, G.: Alcoholism. II. Sex, socioeconomic

status and race in two hospitalized samples, Quarterly Journal of Studies on Alcohol **32**:942, 1971.

33. Robins, L., et al.: Drinking behavior of young urban Negro men. Unpublished paper presented to the joint session of the Annual Meetings of the American Sociological Association and the Society for Study of Social Problems, San Francisco, Aug. 29, 1967.
34. Rosenberg, N., Laessig, R. H., and Rawlings, R. R.: Alcohol, age and fatal traffic accidents, Quarterly Journal of Studies on Alcohol **35**:473, 1974.
35. Rosenblatt, S. M., et al.: Patients admitted for treatment of alcohol withdrawal syndromes, Quarterly Journal of Studies on Alcohol **32**:104, 1971.
36. Schuckit, M. A., and Morrissey, E. R.: Drinking, drinking problems, and "alcoholism" in adolescents. Unpublished paper, 1978.
37. Scott, G.: Blacks in the liquor industry, Black Enterprise **6**:33, 48, 1975.
38. Seto, A., et al.: Biochemical correlates of ethanol-induced flushing in Orientals, Journal of Studies on Alcohol **39**:1, 1978.
39. Simon, W., and Gagnon, J. H.: The end of adolescence: the college experience, New York, 1970, Harper & Row, Publishers.
40. Sterne, M. W.: Drinking patterns and alcoholism among American Negroes. In Pittman, D. J., editor: Alcoholism, New York, 1967, Harper & Row, Publishers.
41. Unger, R. A.: The treatment of adolescent alcoholism, Social Casework **59**:27, 1978.
42. United States Department of Health, Education, and Welfare: A Report on the Indian Health Service Task Force on Alcoholism: alcoholism, a high priority health problem, Publication no. (HSA) 77-1001, Washington, D.C., 1971, Indian Health Service.
43. United States Department of Health, Education, and Welfare: Second special report to the U.S. Congress on alcohol and health, DHEW Publication no. (ADM) 74-124, Washington, D.C., 1978, U.S. Government Printing Office.
44. United States Department of Health, Education, and Welfare: Third special report to the U. S. Congress on alcohol and health, DHEW Publication no. (ADM) 78-569, Washington, D.C., 1978, U.S. Government Printing Office.
45. United States Department of Health, Education, and Welfare: Suicide, homicide and alcoholism among American Indians: guidelines for help, Publication no. (ADM), 74-42, Washington, D.C., 1973, National Institute of Mental Health.
46. United States Department of Health, Education, and Welfare: The unseen crisis: blacks and alcohol, Publication no. (ADM) 17-478, Washington, D.C., 1977, Public Health Service.
47. Wechsler, H., and Thum, D.: Teenage drinking, drug use and social correlates, Quarterly Journal of Studies on Alcohol **34**:1220, 1973.
48. Whitehead, P. C., and Ferrence, R. G.: Alcohol and other drugs related to young drinkers' traffic accident involvement, Journal of Safety Research **8**:65, 1976.
49. Wolff, P. H.: Ethnic differences in alcohol sensitivity, Science **1975**:449, 1972.
50. Wolff, P. H.: Vasomotor sensitivity to alcohol in diverse Mongoloid populations, American Journal of Human Genetics **25**:193, 1973.
51. Young people and alcohol, Alcohol Health and Research World, experimental issue, p. 3, Summer, 1975.
52. Yowell, S., and Brose, C.: Working with drug abuse patients in the ER, American Journal of Nursing **77**:82, 1977.
53. Zeiner, A. R., Paredes, A., and Cowden, L.: Physiologic responses to ethanol among the Tarahumara Indians, Annals of the New York Academy of Sciences **273**:151, 1976.
54. Zeiner, A. R., Paredes, A., and Christensen, H. D.: The role of acetaldehyde in mediating reactivity to an acute dose of ethanol among different racial groups, Alcoholism: Clinical and Experimental Research **3**:11, 1979.

CHAPTER 5

Alcohol problems in special groups
women, the elderly, nurses

The content presented in this chapter is a continuation of the previous one. It provides information about women, the elderly, and nurses with alcohol problems and emphasizes the appraisal process among these special groups.

WOMEN

Until recently researchers studying the effects of alcohol on human behavior have concentrated primarily on the male drinker. Typically, it has been assumed that whatever was learned about male alcoholics could be generalized to women with similar problems. This assumption is currently being challenged, and there is increasing concentration, both in research and treatment efforts, on women with alcoholism. Given the history of this sexual imbalance in alcoholism studies, there still remain many unanswered questions about alcoholism in women, and current findings are sometimes conflicting and not thoroughly substantiated by research. Nevertheless, some findings are becoming clearer, and these will be the emphasis of this section.

Prevalence

Women today are more likely to drink than ever before in history, and the increase is especially true for younger age groups. In addition, female drinkers are developing heavier drinking patterns than in the past, similar to the drinking patterns of men.[6]

It is a large step from drinking to alcoholism, but the number of women alcoholics is also increasing. Conservative estimates of the number of adult women with alcoholism range from 1.5 to 2.25 million or 15% to 22.25% of the total alcoholic population in the United States.[45] When the number of men and women alcoholics is compared, men continue to outnumber women, but the gap is closing.

Reasons for the increase in alcohol use and alcoholism in women are not entirely clear, but changing life-styles and mores most likey have had an effect, since they have led to a redefining of roles for many women. The women's liberation movement has been identified as a factor in the increase in that liberation brings mixed blessings. Women are less bound to the traditional wife-mother role, but as they enter the work world outside the home they are more exposed to hazards typically experienced by men, such as heavier alcoholism rates and early mortality.[1]

There is some evidence, too, that society's attitudes toward alcoholism in women are gradually becoming less negative and punitive. As women feel less guilty about their alcoholism, the need to conceal their drinking diminishes. This factor has led to more accurate identification of numbers of women affected by alcoholism and subsequently to increased research and treatment efforts directed solely at women. It is a hopeful sign for alcoholic women that their problems are finally reaching the attention of workers in the field.

Classification of alcoholic women

Just as there is no typical alcoholic man, there is no typical alcoholic woman representative of all alcoholic women. Alcoholic women come from all segments of society, and their drinking varies not only with the stage of alcoholism but with age, social class, living conditions, and cultural background. Placing them in several general categories, however, is helpful in increasing recognition as to the variations that exist in the total population of women alcoholics. One classification that has been described includes "lace curtain" women, single career women, and skid road women.[15]

The first category, the "lace curtain" woman, includes the secretly imbibing housewife. She has been described so often in movies and novels that she has almost assumed the role of the prototype alcoholic woman in the minds of many. She is typically in her mid-30s to 40s. While her children were growing, she failed to formulate worthwhile goals for herself and used her energies to focus on her children's growth needs and furthering her husband's continued move upward in his career. In her middle years she no longer feels worthwhile or needed. She easily learns that alcohol temporarily removes the ugly feelings of loneliness and depression and therefore she drinks.[15]

A second category includes the single, professional/career woman, who differs considerably from the one just described and may have more in common with her male counterpart. Often she has never married or is divorced or widowed. She may have an interesting, fulfilling job. The problem begins when she returns home at the end of the day and the excitement of the work world is ended. The career woman may have neglected her social life in favor of her business life and only knows how to fill the void during the evening and on weekends with alcohol.[15]

The homeless alcoholic woman has been described as possibly the most socially isolated and disaffiliated member of skid road.[18] Although skid road is a society featuring a great deal of social interaction for the men who live there, for a female inhabitant it is a solitary place. She is far less likely to drink in public places, such as bars or taverns, and even when seen in bars she has limited interactions with others, especially other women. Her contacts with male patrons may be limited to attempts to use sex as a means to continue alcohol consumption. Rooming-house relationships are often short term, but it is easy to find another man and room—at least until she has completely lost her youthful appearance. The latter comes quickly for a skid road woman, largely as a result of her alcohol abuse and life-style.[18]

These categories obviously do not include all female alcoholics, most notably the teenager, women of ethnic minorities, or lesbian women who may use alcohol in unique ways. The categories do provide a broad overview of the variations, alerting one to the need to respond to alcoholic women in an individualized manner.

Special findings
Attitudes toward drunkenness

Alcoholism still carries a greater stigma for women than for men. Although there is apparently a more permissive attitude in American society about social drinking in women, many people continue to view female intoxication with disgust and scorn. Drunkenness in men, on the other hand, is often looked on with indifference, amusement, or pity.[21]

The rejection of female inxotication involves at least two aspects, one relating to the division of labor between the sexes and the other relating to the loss of customary sexual inhibitions and restraints.[25] In the woman's traditional housework role, high levels of skill are not required and moderate degrees of intoxication are not particularly incapacitating. The aspect of a woman's work that is impaired by alcohol intake is the quality of her sensitivity to the needs of others in her roles as wife, mother, daughter, sister, or nursemaid. For example, a drunken mother is incapable of being consistently responsive to the needs of a young child. This factor alone makes drunkenness in women more threatening than in men. The second issue, loss of customary sexual restraints in an intoxicated woman, relates to the historic position noted in the Bible and in Roman law that a woman's drinking and sexual irregularities are linked. Although the popular image of the drunken woman and loose sexual morals persists, the fact is that promiscuity is appropriate to only 5% of all women alcoholics. Most of the other 95% complain of diminished interest in sex.[39]

Societal disapproval of female drunkenness may provide a constraint against heavy drinking, thereby conferring some cultural protection against alcoholism in women. At the same time it has no doubt contributed to making it necessary for many women with alcohol-related problems to drink in secret and to delay seeking treatment until the alcoholism process is far advanced.

Depression

Family history data reveal that depressive disorders and alcoholism are closely related illnesses, and this association is most marked in women. When compared with male alcoholics, women alcoholics show a significant increase in the incidence of depression in close female relatives as well as an overall increased incidence of alcoholism in all close relatives. At the same time women alcoholics themselves are more likely to have depression, whereas alcoholic men are more likely to be sociopathic.[38] The reasons for these differences are unclear, but they may be a result of the contrasting ways in which females and males are socialized in this society. Females are likely to learn that it is acceptable to express feelings through crying, and they may receive extra attention when they are sad. Males are more likely than females to be taught aggressive responses and rewarded for fighting when frustrated.

Several similarities between alcoholism and depression are readily observable. With both conditions the person displays a dysphoric mood, complains of sadness and of feelings of worthlessness, hopelessness, and helplessness. The risk of suicide is high in both alcoholism and depression and especially so for women alcoholics. The rate of completed suicides among female alcoholics is twenty three times the rate for females in the general population and among males it is twenty two times the population rate.[6]

It is of particular importance in appraising women alcoholics to determine if the alcoholism is a primary condition or secondary to some other problem, most notably depression. Are the depressed affect, feelings of hopelessness, and suicidal ideation seen so often in women alcoholics causative or resultant? In many instances an accurate diagnosis of primary depression cannot be made until the woman has been free of alcohol for some time. Clearly the adequacy of subsequent care will be determined largely on the basis of correct diagnosis.

Precipitating factors

The onset of alcoholism and heavy drinking in women has been repeatedly linked to psychologic stress and to some specific precipitating circumstances. Social, environmental, and gynecologic circumstances such as death of a parent or spouse, divorce, hysterectomy, or menopause have been thought to play a special role in the origin of alcoholism in women.[10, 29] One study found that twice as many women as men cited a specific past experience as the point when they started drinking.[29] However, the findings of a more recent study done on heterogeneous sample of 191 women seen at a detoxification center differed from the earlier studies.[32] An evaluation of the time relationship between a number of life stresses and the onset of alcoholism did *not* support the hypothesized tendency of female alcoholics to begin drinking in response to stressful situations. In this study women were asked about their history of alcohol problems and their gynecologic and family histories in separate sections of the interview so that the relationship between the problems would be less likely due to the women's reconstruction of events. Since excessive drinking produces a guilt complex for women, they greatly need an acceptable reason for drinking. Earlier researchers may have made it easy for subjects to state a reason by the sequencing of questions. Whether, in fact, women are more likely than men to develop alcoholism in response to stress awaits further definitive investigation in which men and women alcoholics are compared on similar dimensions.

Once heavy drinking begins to be problematic for a woman, the course into alcoholism tends to be severe and rapid. This generally shortened developmental period of alcoholism in women has been referred to as a "telescoped" effect,[1] leading to the view by some that alcoholism in women is a more virulent process than alcoholism in men.

Multidrug use

Women, in general, exceed men in their consumption of prescribed psychotropic drugs.[8,11] The excessive use of prescription drugs by women in the United States would appear to be related to several factors. Women engage in help-seeking behavior more readily than men, and they tend to describe their symptoms in emotional or psychologic terms. They report feeling worried, tense, or having insomnia, whereas men are more likely to seek help for physical pain. Therefore when women bring their complaints to their physicians, they are more likely than men to receive prescriptions for minor tranquilizers such as diazepam (Valium) and chlordiazepoxide (Librium). Women expect and accept these prescriptions, believing the cultural stereotype that they need psychoactive medications for relief of emotional discomfort associated with aspects of womanhood, such as menstruation, pregnancy, and menopause.

An additional factor sometimes leading to excessive use of prescription drugs by women has to do with myths and misconceptions regarding women still endemic in much of medical education, where the majority of educators are male.[23] For example, it is often taught in medical schools that patients with psychogenic problems are likely to be women. Compounding this is the fact that pharmaceutical advertisements and literature, readily available to medical practitioners, often convey negative attitudes toward female patients and promote the use of psychoactive drugs to treat symptoms common to women.[34] With such influences some male physicians may find it difficult to be objective in their approach to female patients.

The evidence is that women alcoholics use drugs other than alcohol more than men alcoholics do, and as a result multiple dependencies on alcohol and other drugs (predominantly those legally prescribed by physicians) are increasing for women. A major concern in this behalf, as yet little known by professional workers and the general public, has to do with how alcohol interacts with other drugs. Alcohol, when taken in conjunction with other psychoactive drugs, has an additive effect so that it is possible to take a low dose of alcohol and a low dose of chlordiazepoxide (Librium), for example, and together get the effect of taking a large dose. The combination of intoxication, common to alcoholic women, and the ingestion of a psychoactive drug can lead to unintentional overdose resulting in coma or death.

An additional factor of importance for women with multidrug addictions is that they require a longer time to detoxify. It may take up to 2 weeks of detoxification to achieve a drug-free state before referral to a structured rehabilitation program can be made.[15]

The increasing problem of multidrug addictions among women needs to be confronted on several levels. Educational programs need to be launched to inform consumers and prescribers of drugs about the dangers involved in mixing alcohol and other drugs. Women, especially, must become knowledgeable about drug interactions and take special note of their help-seeking behavior with the goal of learning to expect and accept remedies other than drugs for symptoms. When indicated, physicians need to alter their beliefs and understandings about women, and pharmaceutical agencies need to make certain their advertisements are unbiased toward women. Finally, a variety of treatment options need to be provided to all women seeking relief of distressing symptoms.

Biological factors

A larger proportion of women than men suffer from cirrhosis associated with heavy drinking, and women alcoholics, on the average, die at an earlier age—48.6 years as opposed to 56.3 years for men.[48] It has also been shown that women appear to develop cirrhosis at a lower level of alcohol intake and after a shorter duration of excessive drinking.[26, 33]

Another biologic factor of consequence to women alcoholics is that the same dose of alcohol, corrected for body weight, apparently produces higher blood alcohol levels in women than in men.[6] Additionally, blood alcohol levels have been found to vary at different times during the menstrual cycle. The relationship between hormonal balance, menstrual cycle, and alcoholism in women needs further clarification, since current research on the subject is not definitive.

Psychosocial factors

There is evidence that alcoholic persons have a poor self-image and low self-esteem, and this tendency seems to be more pronounced in women than in men.[52] It appears that being alcoholic and a woman is a double jeopardy in American society. Related to this sense of inadequacy is the difficulty many alcoholic women experience with regard to feminine role identity. It has been shown that some women alcoholics wish to be feminine, but their unconscious sex-role confusion causes them to feel somehow inadequate as women.[51] The doubts of the woman alcoholic may be increased by acute threats to her sense of feminine adequacy resulting from experiences such as marital problems, hysterectomy, or children leaving home. When alcohol is used to gain feelings of womanliness, the typical consequences of heavy drinking—neglect of appearance, disapproval by family—eventually make the woman feel less feminine; thus, the proverbial vicious circle is set in motion.

In regard to psychosocial aspects of family life, alcoholic women marry to the same extent but have higher divorce rates than the general population.[21] They are far more likely than alcoholic men to have an alcoholic spouse. The man married to the alcoholic woman is a relatively unknown entity. He has received little research concentration in contrast to his female counterpart and has received more sympathy than censure.[28] Clinical impressions in the literature indicate that the husband of the alcoholic woman reacts to her alcoholism in several ways. He may deny her problem, attempt to control her drinking, or abandon her by actions such as divorce.[14] Men, in particular, need help in comprehending and dealing constructively with an alcohol problem in their spouses. A useful book for assisting them in this process is available.[12] Women married to alcoholic men are less likely to divorce their husbands and struggle for long periods to make their marriages work.

Women alcoholics, as a rule, have experienced more traumatic and disruptive events in their early lives than a normal population and to a greater extent than male alcoholics.[21] The events include having an alcoholic parent, losing a parent through divorce, death, or desertion, and psychiatric illness in the family of origin. The deprivations of childhood may contribute to the alcoholic women's intense search for love and reassurance through marriage and motherhood. When her relationships with people significant to her falter, she is especially vulnerable to the ravages of excessive drinking.

The alcoholic mother

The deleterious effects of an alcoholic mother on her children are undoubtedly manifold. One effect, difficult to measure, has to do with the kind and degree of social, physical, and emotional deprivation children with alcoholic mothers experience. Alcoholic mothers are likely to neglect their children because of preoccupation with alcohol intake and its effects, including intoxication and hangovers.

The offspring of chronic alcoholic women are at risk for developing fetal alcohol syndrome (FAS), caused by the effects of alcohol on the developing fetus. The severity of fetal alcohol syndrome is related to dosage, timing, and individual fetal response. The damage, severe or mild, is irreversible.

Children with full-blown fetal alcohol syndrome exhibit four main categories of abnormalities: (1) central nervous system dysfunctions resulting in varying degrees of mental deficiency or developmental delay; (2) growth deficiencies exhibited by smaller heads than normal and smaller heights and weights, both prenatal and postnatal; (3) characteristic cluster of facial anomalies such as short palpebral fissures (eye slits), thinned upper vermilion (lip), absence or near absence of the philtrum (vertical ridges between nose and upper lip) and epicanthal (eyelid) folds; and (4) variable major and minor malformations, such as heart defects, minor abnormalities of the joints, and external anomalies.[7]

Although fetal alcohol syndrome is more often associated with alcoholism, the effects of moderate levels of alcohol intake during pregnancy are still being investigated. The U.S. Department of Health, Education, and Welfare issued a health caution statement to the general public in mid-1977, describing the potential effects on the fetus of heavy use of alcohol during pregnancy. The statement also said that safe levels of drinking for pregnant women are unknown, but it appears that a risk is established with ingestion above 3 ounces of absolute alcohol, or 6 drinks a day. For intakes of 1 and 3 ounces a day there is still uncertainty but caution is advised.

Given the uncertainty regarding safe levels of alcohol during pregnancy, the wisest decision for a woman anticipating pregnancy is to refrain from all alcohol intake prior to conception and through delivery. The danger of becoming pregnant and not knowing it for a period of several weeks makes cessation of alcohol of importance prior to conception. The anguish of giving birth to a child with fetal alcohol syndrome is difficult to comprehend. Raising a child with this syndrome would present an almost overwhelming challenge to the healthiest of parents. Such an event only compounds the already problem-laden life of the alcoholic woman, promotes the waste of human life, and must be prevented whenever possible. When prevention efforts fail, the option of terminating a pregnancy needs to be made available.

Approaches in appraisal

There are numerous opportunities within health care systems to recognize and treat women with alcohol problems and/or multiple addictions. Nurses need to capitalize on such opportunities and be creative in their efforts to educate and assess involved women. A high index of suspicion for alcohol problems in general and for polydrug abuse and depression in particular is necessary in every contact with a woman seeking help for health purposes. Women clients rarely state alcoholism as their presenting complaint or spontaneously admit to such difficulties. Being continuously mindful that women are especially at risk for the problems cited, the nurse needs to ask female clients specific questions about their drug and alcohol use and be persistent in this questioning until a clear picture of use or nonuse is established.

Before delving into a woman's history regarding alcohol and drug use, it is essential for the nurse to understand her own attitudes about women in general. There are many cultural assumptions about women that, if believed by the nurse, may interfere with accurate appraisal. Consider the following: A woman's prime role is to be a wife and mother, her place is in the home nurturing her husband and children, and to be considered mentally healthy she needs to be submissive, dependent, sensitive, and unassertive. As long as such one-dimensional views about women prevail in health care settings, her care is likely to be laden with biases.

Furthermore, it is of special importance for nurses to scrutinize their beliefs about women and alcoholism carefully. Attitudes of disdain and disgust toward women with alcoholism are still common. The special needs of women alcoholics are ignored too often or indiscriminately lumped with those of men. Such an approach is likely to lead to inept and inaccurate appraisal and to the selection of inappropriate management strategies. Possessing accurate and thorough knowledge about alcoholism in women and having attitudes of empathy and understanding are absolute prerequisites to meaningful involvement with women alcoholics.

The nurse can anticipate that most women alcoholics will feel intimidated during initial interviews. The woman alcoholic's view of herself will no doubt be negative and, as a result of her socialization, she is likely to be submissive and compliant in response to a professional person. The nurse's goal for every contact with the alcoholic woman is to encourage her to take a collaborative role in defining her health problems and in assuming appropriate responsibility for achieving satisfactory resolution of her difficulties. It is essential to allow the alcoholic woman to focus on herself without feeling guilty and to assist her to develop goals directed toward meeting her own needs as well as those of her family. It is also important to be sensitive to a woman's unique capacity to blame herself for almost everything that happens. Asking questions that require the woman to go beyond self-blame is important, such as those which encourage her to see some of her dilemmas in terms of social obstacles. For example, it is especially common for a woman to delay seeking help for a drinking problem. How much of the delay is the responsibility of the woman herself and how much can accurately be attributed to the influences of others who may have assisted her in denying the problem because of the stigma that society places on alcoholism in women? Keeping an appropriate balance between individual painful life experiences and social obstacles is an important challenge for the nurse in appraising the alcoholic woman.

Realizing the importance of family members and close friends in the lives of most alcoholic women, the nurse needs to include these persons, whenever feasible, in appraisal interviews. The woman needs to be reunited in most instances with her family rather than further isolated from them. The constructive involvement of her family can be an essential part of the healing process for the alcoholic woman.

Finally, many alcoholic women are overwhelmed with "shoulds," such as "I should be a good mother," "I should be an outstanding wife," or "I should act in a way to please others." They often need guidance in learning to state their feelings openly and constructively and assistance in finding their own identity. An excellent time to start this process is in the initial contact when appraisal takes place.

Early identification and treatment

Effective means of identifying alcoholism in female populations need to be developed in every setting where women seek health care. Early identification and intervention when alcohol problems are barely beginning are an essential means of assuring full recovery for the majority of afflicted women. Health care personnel need to have a high index of suspicion about the possibility of a female client having an alcohol problem. Additionally, every person working in the area of health care of women needs sound knowledge about female alcoholism, optimistic attitudes toward it, and skill in responding to the special needs of female alcoholic clients. This goal has yet to be fully achieved in the ranks of professional health care workers. Educators of nurses and physicians, for example, have a great responsibility to see that curricula in their institutions of learning are adequate to achieve this goal.

For alcoholism treatment to be truly effective, the unique needs of women must be taken into account. When it is determined that a woman alcoholic needs inpatient treatment, the next obstacle to overcome will often be that of finding adequate care for her children during this period of enforced absence from them. Failure to provide this assistance will keep many women alcoholics from entering agencies for treatment of their alcoholism.

When the typical female alcoholic is admitted to a treatment program, she most likely is experiencing massively diminished self-esteem, is physically debilitated, and is feeling greatly depressed and perhaps suicidal. She is often already divorced or faced with prospects of divorce, has experienced little genuine success in the mothering role, is doubtful she will ever recover from alcoholism, and even if she were to get better has few if any skills for becoming gainfully employed. Innovative techniques that address her special needs are essential to turn her life in the direction of self-confidence and success. The woman alcoholic requires involvement in treatment modalities that will develop her ability to be assertive, enable her to increase her parenting skills, enable her to become confident about being a woman, and cultivate her vocational talents. It is not enough for the woman alcoholic to be simply taught about alcohol and its effect and advised to stay sober. She will need help to discover better ways of coping with life and direction in developing new and varied interests. In many instances she will need treatment for depression and polydrug abuse. In every instance the woman alcoholic will profit from interactions with other women who feel confident about themselves and who are able to provide a role model of women coping successfully with life without using alcohol and other drugs. In a profession such as nursing where the majority of members are female, the healthy, well-educated nurse is among the most qualified of workers to provide the woman alcoholic with a relationship and a rehabilitative environment that holds the promise of full recovery from alcoholism.

ELDERLY PEOPLE

Recognition of a significant problem with alcohol among people in older age groups is of relatively recent origin. In general, alcohol consumption tends to decrease with advancing age. Recent surveys, however, indicate that there are a substantial number of elderly persons who consume enough alcohol to develop alcohol-related problems, and some show signs of alcoholism.[45] Hence, advancing age, contrary to some beliefs, is not a time of life spared from alcoholism.

Old age, it has been said, could be the best time a person ever had. At that time of life one is freed from the task of making a living, from the anxieties of losing a job, and from the need to please superiors to be promoted. One is free to make living one's main business.[16] And yet, the elderly person often is plagued by feelings of worthlessness, emptiness, loneliness, and depression. In addition, deterioration of physical health, loss of family and friends, and limited financial resources, especially with current inflationary trends and fixed incomes, add to existing burdens. If alcohol is used to counteract such stresses, new problems may emerge that compound existing ones and, in some persons, lead to alcoholism.

Elderly persons come to the attention of nurses in hospitals, nursing homes, outpatient clinics, as well as in the privacy of their homes, usually for health concerns of an acute or chronic nature. Unless the nurse is alert to the possible existence of alcoholism in elderly people, the detection of such problems is less likely to occur and the implementation of appropriate corrective actions may never be achieved.

Prevalence

It has been estimated that 10% of persons 60 years of age and over may be alcoholic.[40] This represents approximately 1.6 million persons of the nation's population. As the ratio of elderly in the total population increases, which is expected, so will the number of alcoholics in this age group.

Elderly alcoholic people are most often white (86% to 90% in older people compared with 70% of younger alcoholics), and their rates of separation and divorce are lower than those of younger alcoholics. They tend to live alone.[42]

Although exact figures for the prevalence of alcoholism among elderly women are not available, it has been reported that women have slightly lower percentages of alcoholism than their male counterparts.[44] Related to the greater longevity of women is the finding that the predominence of men alcoholics over women appears to recede in later years; thus there is a greater chance of encountering drinking problems in women than men.[36]

Since alcoholism often coexists with, and not infrequently is the basis for, other health problems, the elderly alcoholic may come to the attention of health care providers as a client in health care or social agencies. Studies of general hospital admissions, for instance, showed that 18% to 56% of elderly medical admissions and 23% of psychiatric admissions were persons with alcoholism.[30, 42, 47] Thirteen percent of patients of a medical home care program and 12% of elderly persons of a psychiatric outpatient program were noted to be alcoholic, indicating that alcoholism in the elderly is indeed a substantial problem.[2,42]

Diagnosis

Alcohol problems in reference to the elderly are used throughout this discussion to designate impairment in physical or mental health or threat to the social stability of the person, as a consequence of alcohol consumption. Alcoholism is used to mean the presence of physical dependence on alcohol and/or the existence of alcohol-related conditions that are rated as major indicators of alcoholism in the *Criteria for the Diagnosis of Alcoholism,* described in Chapter 2.[9]

There is no doubt that alcohol problems compound the stresses of old age and that recognition, identification, and interventions are essential to improve the quality of life among the elderly. Yet obstacles to the identification of alcohol problems remain.

Diagnosing alcoholism in elderly persons is more difficult than it is in younger persons for several reasons. There is generally a low awareness among health care professionals regarding the possibility of alcoholism in the elderly. Alcoholism is simply not suspected. Even in the presence of obvious alcohol-related symptoms, the diagnosis may be missed. At times nurses recognize symptoms of alcoholism, yet feel unprepared to intervene knowledgeably. In one study of 50 male patients 65 years of age and over, more than half the diagnoses missed in patients on medical or surgical wards were either alcoholism or depression. In another study no mention of alcohol or drug-related problems was made for 17 patients who had positive scores on a test, indicating the existence of alcoholism.[43, 49] Knowledge of alcoholism, its symptoms, and progression coupled with interpersonal skills and accepting attitudes by nurses are essential to identify and help the elderly alcoholic.

Another obstacle hampering diagnosis is related to shielding of the alcoholic person by members of his family or close friends. Family members will go to great efforts to hide the elderly person's drinking practices and to deny the existence of a drinking problem. To the family it is unthinkable that grandmother or grandfather has a problem with alcohol. The continued prevalence of social rejection of the alcoholic person and views of sinful behavior connected with alcohol abuse tend to perpetuate maneuvers that prevent the detection of alcoholism. Even if the alcoholic person recognizes the existence of alcoholism, he refrains from seeking help for fear of censure by loved ones and friends, and especially for fear of losing the use of alcohol. At times alcoholism remains unrecognized because the quantity of alcohol consumed by the elderly is not always a useful indicator of its consequences. Even relatively moderate amounts of alcohol may have serious effects on behavioral and physiologic functions.

The diagnosis of alcoholism in the elderly is further complicated by the fact that diagnostic criteria have been established for use with middle-aged populations and therefore may not be appropriate for older people. For instance, signs of physical addiction, such as tremors and minimal disorientation, may be ongoing conditions in the elderly. Furthermore, alcohol may cause problems to the person without its progressing to physical dependence. Symptoms of confusion, staggering gait, drowsiness, listlessness, and uncommunicativeness should lead to assessment of possible alcohol problems. Quantity-frequency measurements of alcohol use require comparisons with normal drinking, and measurements of normal drinking practices for the elderly are not available. It is known that quantity and frequency of drinking change with age, and even minimal drinking may have implications for health in the elderly.[5]

Health problems in the elderly may compound the recognition of alcohol problems. Degenerative diseases and psychopathologic conditions can mimic symptoms of alcoholism. General deterioration, malnutrition, mental deterioration, domestic quarrels, and social isolation may easily be ascribed to the effects of age rather than to the consequence of heavy drinking. Careful appraisal will help clarify the etiology of symptomatology.

In diagnosing alcoholism among the elderly, two rather distinct groupings are recognized.[53] One group of persons have been drinking heavily for many years and have survived to old age. This group is remarkable in itself, since heavy drinking tends to decline with advancing age and premature death from alcoholism generally prevents living to old age. It has been reported that younger alcoholics who do reach an older age generally stop drinking after a mean of twenty years of alcohol intake and demonstrate about eleven years of abstinence.[42] It is estimated that this "early onset" group represents about two thirds of elderly alcoholics. Persons in this group seem to have personality characteristics similar to those of younger alcoholics.[53]

The second group of elderly persons, called "late-onset" group, represents those who developed their alcoholism later in life, most likely in response to depression, bereavement, retirement, loneliness, or physical illness.[53] Since their alcoholism is of shorter duration, physiologic consequences tend to be less severe, and treatment efforts are often more effective.

Causative factors

What causes alcoholism in the elderly? As is true for people in younger age groups, whether or not alcoholism develops probably depends on multiple factors, including the interaction of genetic predispositions, the level of stresses encountered, and the character of existing coping mechanisms.[22,41]

The stresses of advancing age are multiple and often difficult to manage. Retirement requires adjustment to a new way of life. There is often bereavement and depression resulting from the loss of loved ones, with subsequent social isolation and loneliness. Physical deterioration further adds to the pressures as the zest for life and the energy to carry on decrease. The use of alcohol constitutes one of the remaining pleasures that makes life tolerable. In the presence of genetic predisposition, persons using alcohol to cope with stresses may go on to develop alcoholism. An additional contributing factor is a decrease in tolerance to alcohol, which has been reported by older people as well as by many chronic alcoholics.[19] The person experiences the effects of alcohol in relatively small doses so that even moderate alcohol consumption can lead to alcohol problems. This may be partly due to differences in metabolism of alcohol in older people or, as has been noted recently, to a smaller volume of body water and a decrease in lean body tissue in older people.[37,48a]

Following is an account by a 71-year-old man:

I have always liked my drink and I have always been a very active man, but since I have been getting older, the "oomph" and the zest for life have gradually been going, and the desire to get on with my job (on the farm) is getting less. My work is optional; I am my own boss, but I have a sense of guilt if I do not get out to work. A drink in the morning helps me to get out of bed and out on the farm. Anyway, I doubt that I drink more than previously, but what I drink now affects me much more than before.*

Symptoms of alcohol problems

What then are indicators or symptoms that must alert the nurse to the possible existence of alcohol problems in a nursing appraisal of the elderly person? Many of the symptoms applicable to the diagnosis of alcoholism in general populations can also be recognized in the elderly person, such as puffiness around the eyes and the odor of alcohol on the breath. Changes discussed below are those more often associated with elderly alcoholics.

In general, it is important to note that the manifestations of alcoholism in the elderly are more subtle than in younger persons, and greater efforts are required to elicit the presence of problems associated with alcohol consumption.[53] This may be true in part because when the elderly person consumes alcohol, he displays a striking lack of awareness to associated impairments.[4] In addition, intentional distortions and the phenomenon of "blackouts" may make self-report information inaccurate, necessitating careful questioning and, when possible, obtainment of data from more reliable sources such as family members.

In the course of history taking when the incidence of accidents appears greater than would be expected, suspicion of alcohol overuse should be aroused. In a public project, elderly tenants were observed to have many head and leg injuries from falls and fatalities from fires.[31] An investigation led to the identification of alcohol problems in many of the tenants and ultimately to steps dealing with these problems. Likewise, falls leading to fractures were observed to be common occurrences in a nursing home setting and were related to excessive drinking.[20] Bruises on legs caused by bumping into furniture are observed more frequently in elderly than in younger persons because of the effects of intoxication coupled with declining motor skills.

Elderly alcoholics show an increase in various health problems. In a study of 55 elderly hospitalized alcoholics a significantly higher rate of physiologic symptoms rated as severe, such as hematemesis and hematuria, existed compared with a nonalcoholic cohort.[17] In another study a specific health problem occurring with greater frequency in elderly alcoholics than in a younger group was that of chronic obstructive lung disease. Since elderly alcoholic persons also were observed to be heavy smokers, the presence of lung problem was not surprising.[42]

---

*From Glatt, M. M.: Experiences with elderly alcoholics in England, Alcoholism: Clinical and Experimental Research **2**:23-26, 1978. By permission.

Tremulousness, although possibly an indicator of some coexisting illness, should arouse suspicion of increased alcohol consumption. The elderly person who jokes about needing help with his bath or having difficulty when brushing his teeth may drink too much.

Occasionally the diagnosis of alcoholism is made on the appearance of symptoms caused by sudden withdrawal of alcohol. These may show as severe tremulousness, hallucinations, seizure activity, or delirium tremens, the latter characterized by an acute confusional state. Confusion may also be a function of arteriosclerotic brain disease, a sign of intoxication, or a symptom of Wernicke's encephalopathy. An alcohol withdrawal reaction was reported in an 80-year-old woman who became confused after surgery. She had brought a stock of liquor with her to the hospital but was unable to reach the bottles because of her physical incapacity.[36]

Malnutrition in an elderly person may be an indicator of alcohol overuse, and the nurse should investigate its existence. The elderly person who shows changes in weight, notably loss of weight, changes in appetite, abdominal distress, vomiting, or altered bowel habits may satisfy caloric intake by using alcohol rather than food. Nutritional deficiencies may subsequently lead to vitamin deficiencies, blood dyscrasias, and behavioral disturbances.

Unexpected or untoward effects of drugs may result from the concomitant intake of alcohol and other drugs. Alcohol interacts with many other drugs, affecting their absorption, metabolism, storage, and utilization. In the elderly, alcohol combined with prescription drugs such as tranquilizers, antihypertensive agents, anticoagulants, digitalis, diuretics, insulin, or iron preparations is of particular concern. When alcohol is used in addition to prescription drugs, the potential for psychophysiologic disturbances is intensified. Definitive information on alcohol and drug interactions is presented in Chapter 6, Table 4. Meticulous appraisal as to kinds and amounts of drugs the person is using is an essential prerequisite to the prevention of serious consequences.

Social isolation may be a distinct indicator of alcohol overuse. The elderly person who watches television all day and drinks as he watches in preference to interacting with people is suspect for alcohol abuse. In a recent study, elderly alcoholics reported minimal social participation when compared with elderly nonalcoholic persons. This was most pronounced with respect to sharing of personal life experiences with others, such as close friends and relatives.[35] Those who have lost family and friends feel loneliness even more acutely. Alienation, which has been related to increased drinking, was found to be greater in elderly problem drinkers than in other age cohorts.[35] Bereavement, an important cause of depression in middle and late life, also may precipitate excessive drinking.

Approaches in appraisal

When an attempt is made to identify alcoholism in an elderly person, assessing the reasons for drinking may be extremely important. Suspicion of a problem with alcohol should be aroused when loneliness, anxiety, grief, depression, dull physical pain or lack of anything else to do are given as reasons for drinking. Drinking for social integration, on the other hand, may be a more healthy indicator of alcohol use for some elderly people.

Alertness to the possibility of alcohol problems in the elderly and knowledge of what to look for and how to evaluate presenting problems are important elements of the appraisal process. Of equal or perhaps even greater importance in communicating with the elderly is the nurse's sensitivity to their special needs and problems. The quality of the relationship that ensues depends partly on this sensitivity.

Communication is of central importance in any human behavior. Orderly communication between people generally leads to adaptive behaviors, whereas disordered communication, such as misunderstandings, can lead to maladaptive behavior patterns of frustration and anger.[3] To understand that elderly persons have unique characteristics and to take these into account when relating to them will enhance communications.

As a person gets older, changes are likely to occur in perceptions about self and in the acuity of senses. Feelings of self-worth decrease as a consequence of multiple interactive events. With the relinquishing of a job and as all relationships decrease, sources from which information about one's competencies are generally obtained diminish. At the same time decreases in sensory perceptions engender feelings of insecurity and vulnerability. Such feelings are further intensified in the presence of alcoholism, and the afflicted person may feel of little worth. The nurse, in her relationship with the elderly person, can work toward counteracting such feelings by approaching the person with dignity and respect and encouraging him to make choices and decisions. This enables him to experience a feeling of power to direct his own life. Such a relationship can do much to increase the elderly person's self-worth.

Hearing loss and visual deficits are among the most common sensory changes in the elderly. Some simple techniques carried out by the nurse enhance communication, such as positioning herself so that it is possible to reach out and touch the person. Chairs should be of the same height. Speaking clearly, slowly, and using appropriate language convey a sense of interest and importance and of wanting to be understood. Pacing the interview so that the elderly person has ample time to respond is of particular importance when talking with an elderly alcoholic person, since it may be difficult for him to recall recent events. Being responsive to nonverbal clues, such as facial expressions, gestures, and postures is likely to aid the information-gathering process. The use of touch is a highly appropriate means of conveying warmth and making contact, and as a rule elderly people are less inhibited about touch than are young persons and respond to it positively.[3] All these approaches tend to contribute to a more effective appraisal of the elderly person. At the same time it is important to remember that approaches must be individualized. Not every elderly person has sensory deficits, nor do they all have feelings of low self-worth. To anticipate some of the aforementioned problems helps the nurse to be prepared to meet situations with skill and competence. Yet this must never preclude an individualized appraisal.

Prevention and treatment

Preventing alcohol problems in the elderly is synonymous with a concern for the fulfillment of each person's basic human needs and rights. Responding to loneliness and the need for love, providing an environment for activity and self-actualization, respecting a person for what he is, and relating to him in a dignified and respectful manner promote feelings of worth and well-being. If such conditions prevail the overuse of alcohol is less likely to occur.

The treatment of alcoholism in the elderly rests on the same principles as does treatment for other age groups. Alcohol intake must be restricted or stopped, depending on the seriousness of the condition, the absence or presence of physical dependence, or both. In the presence of the latter, complete abstinence may be the only possible goal for rehabilitation.

Nursing appraisal of the person's total situation, including psychosocial and physiologic states with subsequent identification of major problems, must be addressed. The findings of the appraisal interview need to be shared with the client and, with his participation, management strategies need to be identified and implemented.

In general, elderly persons whose alcoholism is of recent origin tend to respond well to therapeutic interventions. They are more likely to remain in treatment and they benefit, in particular, from social and interpersonal types of interventions. Furthermore, the natural decline of the desire for alcohol that usually accompanies advancing age favors interventive approaches.

Those persons who began drinking early in life and continued to drink excessively into old age have a less favorable prognosis. Even they, however, will show improvement when abstinence from drinking is achieved and other life problems are addressed.

For the elderly, issues in obtaining health care services relate to insufficient money, distance from health providers and care agencies, and the often prevailing attitude among health professionals that not much can be done to improve the health of elderly persons. All of these conditions can be changed. With manipulation of the environment, the provision of social support, and the improvement of general conditions of health, the elderly person's alcohol problems can be halted and he can be helped to live in comfort and satisfaction.

NURSES

It may seem inconceivable to many nurses that one of their professional colleagues could be an alcoholic. Yet it has been estimated that as many as 40,000 nurses in the United States have alcoholism.[24] With such a large number of afflicted nurses, it is almost certain that at some time in her career every nurse will have close association with an alcoholic nurse colleague.

Since the majority of nurses have had little or no formal education about alcoholism, most are ill prepared to recognize and respond constructively to the problem when it arises in their professional ranks. Lacking knowledge and no doubt feeling the great stigma attached to alcoholism, especially in women, many nurses either ignore the problem in a colleague, make excuses, or assign reasons other than drinking to the symptoms. None of these responses is helpful. They are of no value to the nurse with the drinking problem, to the patients she serves, or to the overall morale and productivity of the unit where the nurse is employed. Although it is common to feel helpless and confused when faced with a colleague who has drinking problems, such feelings can be erased with the acquisition of knowledge and skill. It is essential that nurses learn the clues indicating a colleague may have a drinking problem and that they become competent in their ability to motivate the drinker into treatment long before alcoholism is advanced.

Clues

As a rule, alcoholism is an insidious process, and the nurse may continue producing excellent work on the job for a period of time in spite of heavy drinking. (A personal account of how alcoholism affected the private and professional life of one nurse is described in a forthright manner in an article by Schnurr.[46]) As alcohol consumption increases, overt symptoms make their appearance. The clues found in the list below are frequently occurring behaviors in the actively employed nurse with a drinking problem. In addition, the alcoholic nurse can be expected to demonstrate other stigmata of alcoholism as described in Chapters 2 and 3. Clues to drug abuse other than alcohol in nurses are also available.[13]

Frequent use of sick leave, often coinciding with days off
Lateness for work
Failure to return from lunch break or disappearing in the middle of a shift
Irritability with patients and staff
Sleeping or dozing on the job

Use of other drugs, especially amphetamines and minor tranquilizers, sometimes
    acquired from unit medication supply
Withdrawal from others
Deterioration in work habits
    Careless charting
    Illegible handwriting
    Patient care errors, such as administering wrong medication
    Shunning of extra work assignments
    Forgetfulness
Complaints from staff and patients about lack of quality and quantity of work
Alcohol on breath on the job
Drinking, in isolated spot, on the job
Shakiness

Frequently the manner of behaving will represent a departure from the nurse's usual mode of conduct. It has been found, for example, that many alcoholic nurses have been in the top one third of their classes, attained advanced degrees, and held demanding, responsible positions functioning with a high level of competence. They have tended to be particularly ambitious, achievement-oriented nurses before succumbing to the effects of alcoholism.[24] For these reasons a nurse who changes from a highly functional state to a deteriorating one will be especially noticeable to co-workers.

Confrontation

When it is evident that a nurse's ability to function on the job is impaired, for whatever reason, it is necessary that she be confronted about her job performance. Most units where nurses work have mechanisms for periodically undertaking systematic evaluation of workers, with specific people designated to accomplish the task. If a staff nurse, for example, is suspected of having an alcohol problem, it is the responsibility of co-workers to speak directly with the nurse in charge about their observations. The observations shared need to be specific instances of poor job performance rather than general statements about their suspicions that the staff nurse drinks too much. Many times nurses fail to take this important step because they fear reprisal or they are concerned about getting a friend in trouble. Nurses need to understand, however, that failure to share observations with appropriate people about the deteriorating job performance of an alcoholic colleague is to withhold crucial information. Only when the colleague's job performance problems are explicitly identified can they be discussed openly and constructive management instituted.

When the nurse with a drinking problem is a supervisor, it is suggested that concerned nurse subordinates go to the supervisor's superior with specific examples about job performance, especially when it seems the problem is going unnoticed or is escalating.[50] Accomplishing this task in a small group of two or three nurses is often an effective way of sharing a difficult task and of conveying the extent and gravity of the problem. What is important is that observations get reported to appropriate persons regardless of where in the heirarchy the nurse with problems is functioning.

The nurse in charge has the responsibility of carrying out actual confrontation of the employee with job-related problems. This is often a difficult task to accomplish successfully. The purpose of the confrontation is to enable the troubled nurse to begin to acknowledge the reality of deteriorating job performance and to determine what steps to take to correct the problem. It is usually best not to tie the difficulties on the job to alcohol unless there are specific instances, for example, of alcohol use on the job or coming to work with alcohol on the breath. Rather, the charge nurse needs to describe calmly specific incidents where the nurse's work performance was below expectations. The charge nurse might say, "You have been absent from work on four different days during the last month and have left work two hours early on three other days during the same month." Even when the charge nurse conveys genuine concern about the employee's difficulties, it can be expected that the alcoholic nurse will react defensively when confronted with specific incidents. Counterdefensiveness is not helpful and will likely lead to debate or argument about the accuracy of some aspect of the incident. It is best to stay close to factual data and not get involved in emotional exchanges.

Clearly the alcoholic nurse's behavior on the job must change if employment is to continue. This fact needs to be clarified along with achieving agreement as to exactly what needs alteration and the time period for accomplishing the change.

Referral and treatment

It is also the responsibility of the charge nurse to know exactly where to refer the employee for diagnostic evaluation. Being vague or poorly informed about specific telephone numbers or names of agencies provides too much opportunity for a reluctant person to delay getting assistance. Sometimes there are employee assistance programs within the place of employment where the nurse can be referred. More often an off-site facility must be utilized. The latter, a program removed from the work environment, may be more acceptable in some instances to the nurse. It is the responsibility of the counselor within the referral agency to determine the underlying problem and if it is alcoholism, to recommend appropriate action. Sometimes detoxification is needed prior to involvement in a long-term inpatient or outpatient rehabilitation program. Some nurses respond well to Alcoholics Anonymous (AA) and receive all the help they need for recovery there, especially when the AA group consists of other nurses or is predominantly composed of professional persons. On occasion it is possible for the afflicted nurse to continue employment simultaneously with treatment. Others may need varying lengths of leave from the job to effect recovery. Several treatment programs designed specifically for addicted nurses have been described.[24, 27, 50]

When the nurse returns to the job, it will be necessary to monitor her work carefully for at least a year to make certain she is not hazardous in any way to self, patients, and co-workers.[24] Constant surveillance, however, is usually unwarranted and only heightens any anxiety the nurse may have about her ability to do well. The nurse will need periodic feedback about performance to indicate the ways she is achieving according to expectations and to point out and immediately correct any problems that arise. The nurse will need a special measure of support and understanding for a period of time, but this should not be confused with overprotectiveness.

As more and more alcoholic nurses are identified and aided by their colleagues to seek rehabilitation, not only will the afflicted nurses benefit but so will the entire nursing profession. What is done to assist alcoholic nurses is easily transferable to members of allied professional groups who, like nurses, have no immunity to alcoholism.

REFERENCES

1. Alcoholism and women, Alcohol Health and Research World, p. 2, Summer, 1974.
2. Bailey, M. D., Haberman, P. W., and Alksne, H.: The epidemiology of alcohol in an urban residential area, Quarterly Journal of Studies on Alcohol **26**:20, 1965.
3. Blazer, D.: Techniques for communicating with your elderly patient, Geriatrics **11**:79-84, 1978.
4. Blose, I. L.: The relationship of alcohol and aging and the elderly, Alcoholism: Clinical and Experimental Research **2**:17, 1978.
5. Cahalan, D., Cissin, I. H., and Crossley, H. M.: American drinking practices, New Brunswick, N.J., 1960, Rutgers Center of Alcohol Studies.
6. Carrigan, Z. H.: Research issues: women and alcohol abuse, Alcohol Health and Research World **3**:1, 1978.
7. Clarren, S. K., and Smith, D. W.: The fetal alcohol syndrome experience with 65 patients and a review of the world literature, New England Journal of Medicine **19**:1063, 1978.
8. Cooperstock, R.: Women and psychotropic drugs. In MacLennan, A., editor: Women: their use of alcohol and other legal drugs, Toronto, 1976, Addiction Research Foundation of Ontario.
9. Criteria Committee, National Council on Alcoholism: Criteria for the diagnosis of alcoholism, Annals of Internal Medicine **77**:249, 1972; American Journal of Psychiatry **129**:127, 1972.
10. Curlee, J.: Alcoholism and the "empty nest," Bulletin of the Menninger Clinic **33**:165, 1969.
11. Curlee, J.: A comparison of male and female patients at an alcoholism treatment center, Journal of Psychology **74**:239, 1970.
12. Curlee-Salisbury, J.: When the woman you love is an alcoholic, St. Meinrad, Ind., 1978, Abbey Press.
13. Elaine, B., et al.: Helping the nurse who misuses drugs, American Journal of Nursing **74**:1665, 1974.

14. Estes, N. J., and Baker, J.: Spouses of alcoholic women. In Estes, N. J., and Heinemann, M. E., editors: Alcoholism development, consequences and interventions, St. Louis, 1977, The C. V. Mosby Co.
15. Fraser, W.: The alcoholic woman: attitudes and perspectives. In MacLennan, A., editor: Women: their use of alcohol and other legal drugs, Toronto, 1976, Addiction Research Foundation of Ontario.
16. Fromm, E.: The psychological problems of aging. Albany, April, 1967, New York State Executive Department, Office for the Aging (11 N. Pearl St., Albany, N.Y. 12207).
17. Funkhouser, M.: Identifying alcohol problems among elderly hospital patients, Alcohol Health and Research World 2:27, Winter, 1977/1978.
18. Garrett, G. R., and Bahr, H. M.: Women on Skid Row, Quarterly Journal of Studies on Alcohol 34:1228, 1973.
19. Glatt, M. M.: Drinking habits of English (middle class) alcoholics, Acta Psychiatrica Scandinavica 37:38, 1961.
20. Glatt, M. M.: Experiences with elderly alcoholics in England, Alcoholism: Clinical and Experimental Research 2:23, 1978.
21. Gomberg, E.: Women and alcoholism. In Franks, V., and Vansanti, B., editors: Women in therapy—new psychotherapies for a changing society, New York, 1974, Brunner/Mazel, Inc.
22. Goodwin, D.: Is alcoholism hereditary? New York, 1976, Oxford University Press.
23. Howell, M. C.: What medical schools teach about women, the New England Journal of Medicine 291:304, 1974.
24. Isler, C.: The alcoholic nurse: what we try to deny, RN 41:48, July, 1978.
25. Knupfer, G.: Female drinking patterns. Presented at the Fifteenth Annual Meeting of the North American Association of Alcoholism Programs, Washington, D.C., Sept. 1964.
26. Lelbach, W. K.: Organic pathology related to volume and patterns of alcohol use. In Gibbins, R. J., et al., editors: Research advances in alcohol and drug problems, New York, 1974, John Wiley & Sons, Inc.
27. Levine, D., et al.: A special program for nurse addicts, American Journal of Nursing 74:1672, 1974.
28. Lindbeck, L. J.: The woman alcoholic: a review of the literature, International Journal of the Addictions 7:567, 1972.
29. Lisansky, E.: Alcoholism in women: social and psychological concomitants. I. Social history data, Quarterly Journal of Studies on Alcohol 18:588, 1957.
30. McCusker, J., Cherubin, C. E., and Zimberg, S.: Prevalence of alcoholism in general municipal hospital population, New York State Journal of Medicine 71:751, 1971.
31. Mishaps clues to drinking by elderly, NIAAA Information and Feature Service, p. 2, Nov. 2, 1978.
32. Morrissey, E. A., and Schuckit, M.: Stressful life events and alcohol problems among women seen at a detoxification center, Journal of Studies on Alcohol 39:1559, 1978.
33. Pequignot, G., et al.: Increasing risk of liver cirrhosis with intake of alcohol, La Revue De L'Alcolisme 20:191, 1974.
34. Prather, J., and Fidell, L. S.: Sex differences in the content and style of medical advertisement, Social Science and Medicine 9:23, 1975.
35. Rathbone-McCuan, E.: Community survey of aged alcoholics and problem drinkers, Baltimore, June, 1976, Levindale Geriatric Research Center.
36. Rosin, A. J., and Glatt, M. M.: Alcohol excess in the elderly, Quarterly Journal of Studies on Alcohol 32:53, 1971.
37. Salzman, C., van der, Kolk, B., and Shader, R. I.: Psychopharmacology and the geriatric patient. In Shader, R. I., editor: Manual of psychiatric therapeutics, Boston, 1975, Little Brown & Co., Inc.

38. Schuckit, M.: The alcoholic woman: a literature review, Psychiatry in Medicine **3**:37, 1972.
39. Schuckit, M.: Sexual disturbance in the woman alcoholic, Medical Aspects of Human Sexuality **6**:44, 48, 53, 57, 60, 65, 1972.
40. Schuckit, M.: Geriatric alcoholism and drug abuse, Gerontologist **17**:168, 1977.
41. Schuckit, M., Goodwin, D., and Winokur, G.: A study of alcoholism in half siblings, American Journal of Psychiatry **128**:1132, 1972.
42. Schuckit, M., and Miller, P. L.: Alcoholism in elderly men: a survey of general medical ward. In Seixas, F. A., and Eggleston, S., editors: Work in progress in alcoholism, Annals of the New York Academy of Sciences **273**:558-571, 1976.
43. Schuckit, M., Miller, P. D., and Hahlbohm, D.: Unrecognized psychiatric illness in elderly medical-surgical patient, Journal of Gerontology **30**:65, 1975.
44. Schuckit, M., and Pastor, P. A., Jr.: Alcohol-related psychopathology in the aged. In Kaplan, O. J., editor: Psychopathology in the aging, New York, 1979, Academic Press, Inc.
45. Secretary of Health, Education, and Welfare: Third Special Report to the U. S. Congress on alcohol and health, Washington, D.C., 1978, U.S. Government Printing Office.
46. Schnurr, S. E.: The alcoholic professional. Part I. Alcoholism and health, Family and Community Health **2**:33, 1979.
47. Simon, A., Epstein, L. J., and Reynolds, L.: Alcoholism in geriatric mentally ill, Geriatrics **23**:125, 1968.
48. Spain, D. M.: Portal cirrhosis of the liver: a review of 250 necropsies with reference to sex differences, American Journal of Psychiatry **15**:215, 1945.
48a. Vestal, R. E., et al.: Aging and ethanol metabolism, Clinical Pharmacology and Therapeutics **21**:343, 1977.
49. Westermeyer, J.: An assessment of hospital care for the alcoholic patient, Alcoholism: Clinical and Experimental Research **2**:53, 1978.
50. When a colleague's drinking becomes your headache, RN **41**:31, July, 1978.
51. Wilsnack, S.: Femininity by the bottle, Addictions **20**:3, 1973.
52. Wood, H. P., and Duffy, E. L.: Psychological factors in alcoholic women, American Journal of Psychiatry **123**:341, 1966.
53. Zimberg, S.: Diagnosis and treatment of the elderly alcoholic, Alcoholism: Clinical and Experimental Research **2**:27, 1978.

CHAPTER 6

Appraisal by interview
tools and guides

It is a truism that the major portion of the data needed for a complete and accurate health appraisal can be obtained by means of skillful interviewing. The interview conducted prior to the physical examination is used primarily to obtain a health history, to elicit symptoms, and to determine if and how symptoms affect daily living activities. Interviewing skill and knowledge about alcohol and alcoholism must be combined to acquire a thorough data base. Skill alone in interviewing is of little value until the nurse knows the implication of different symptoms of alcoholism so that relevant questions can be posed. At the same time, mere knowledge of the pathology of alcoholism is insufficient for guiding clients to submit maximal information for their own benefit. Skill in interviewing and knowledge of pathology are acquired through study and guided practice, and the two must be integrated concomitantly in appraisal and diagnosis.

The appraisal interview can be utilized for additional purposes beyond the basic one of finding out what is wrong with the client. The nurse who is sensitive to the nuances of a beginning relationship can use the appraisal interview as a vehicle for building trust and understanding—essential ingredients for the initiation and continuation of a therapeutic relationship. During the interview the nurse needs to ascertain the client's perceptions regarding his condition and to consider these perceptions in planning future care. Using knowledge about alcohol and alcoholism, the nurse can listen for myths and misconceptions held by the client about his condition. Thus on occasion the appraisal interview can be used to correct misinformation. This may enable some clients to see their symptomatology, and what to do about it, in a different and more hopeful light. Many alcoholic clients, for example, fear the incurability of alcoholism and delay personal identification with such a diagnosis. It is not unusual for the client to ask during the course of an interview, "Do you think I can make it?" The nurse who is knowledgeable about alcoholism and at ease with the subject can honestly respond, "If you accept that you have a drinking problem and cooperate with treatment, there is every reason to believe you will get better." Such a straightforward response, which places the primary responsibility for recovery with the client, can serve as a powerful motivating device for continued treatment.

For many clients the appraisal interview is a unique experience, since it is the first time they have taken stock of the comprehensive effects of alcohol in all aspects of their lives. Drawing all these data together at one point in time with the aid of an empathic, knowledgeable nurse can provide the stimulus needed to interrupt the destructive cycle of alcoholism and promote the active pursuit of health. Finally, in taking and in giving a complete drinking history, both the nurse and client are desensitized to talking about alcohol, setting the stage for further open discussions around a subject that is too often taboo.

What kinds of tools are useful in obtaining appraisal data by means of interview? The main purpose of this chapter is to describe tools and guides that can be used in appraising for the presence of alcohol-related problems. Screening tools for the general population of persons seen in health care facilities and interview guides for accomplishing immediate and in-depth nursing appraisal of suspected or known alcoholic clients are described.

TOOLS FOR GENERAL APPRAISAL

In American society where alcohol use is commonplace, it is essential to include screening questions for alcohol problems on all persons who come to the attention of health care personnel, regardless of the setting. If the goal of early identification of alcohol problems is ever to be achieved, before symptoms are far advanced, the use of alcoholism screening questions will need to become as routine as questions about diet and smoking. Such screening only takes a few moments, but it does require the nurse to feel at ease talking with people about alcohol and its use and to be knowledgeable about the features of alcoholism.

Direct questions that require factual responses are the most useful in determining the presence of alcohol-related problems. The nurse needs to ask the questions matter-of-factly, along with obtaining answers about other health-related issues. Asking first about other drug usage, such as caffeine and nicotine, and then leading into alcohol provides a less obtrusive pathway for initiating discussion about alcohol use. Following is one set of questions that can be used[20]:

Now I'd like to learn about your use of alcohol.

Do you drink at all?

If yes, has anyone ever said that drinking might be causing a problem for you?

Has your wife (husband) or someone close to you ever complained about your drinking?

How much do you drink on the average?

Have you ever had to consider cutting down on your drinking?

The initial question is posed to discover if the person uses alcohol at all. If the answer is no, it is useful to ask a question or two to clarify the basis for the individual's nonuse. The person may be an abstainer for religious reasons, for example, or because of a prior problem with alcohol—facts the nurse needs to know in planning individualized management strategies. If the person answers affirmatively to the initial question, the next two questions in the set are designed to focus on what another person might be saying about the client's drinking. Frequently it is someone close to the drinker who is the first to be acutely aware of evolving difficulties with alcohol. The fourth question about the amount of alcohol consumed is of importance particularly in regard to the development of tolerance. With tolerance a person is able to consume increasing quantities of alcohol but with less noticeable effect on behavior. Once tolerance has developed, a long "silent" period follows during which the symptoms of alcoholism become entrenched.[14] The final question in the set attempts to uncover if the person has had to try to control his drinking. When answered positively, it separates the social drinker, who does not need to be concerned with such matters, from the person with a developing alcohol problem.

Another useful alcoholism screening tool for use in the general population of clients is the Short Michigan Alcoholism Screening Test (SMAST).[15] The SMAST provides an objective way of screening for alcoholism and can be administered without extensive prior training. The test consists of thirteen questions to be answered "Yes" or "No" either by the person filling in the questionnaire or by the interviewer asking the same questions verbally in interview form. Using the latter method, the interviewer can clarify any questions that the person may have.

To understand the SMAST more fully, it is useful to consider the purpose of the questions.

1. Do you feel you are a normal drinker?
3. Do you ever feel guilty about your drinking?

Questions 1 and 3 ask the person to state how he feels about his drinking in comparison with others and to tell whether he feels blameworthy about it. Many people will deny alcoholism but will admit that their drinking and their response to it in some way differs from most others around them.

2. Does your wife, husband, a parent, or other near relative ever worry or complain about your drinking?
4. Do friends or relatives think you are a normal drinker?
7. Has drinking ever created problems with you and your wife, husband, a parent, or other near relative?

Questions 2, 4, and 7 look for the presence of family problems related to alcohol consumption. Family members, living in close proximity to the drinker, are frequently among the first to notice and to be affected by excessive alcohol use.

5. Are you able to stop drinking when you want to?

Question 5 examines loss of control, a symptom most frequently experienced by the alcoholic person as a lack of control once an episode of drinking has begun. Forces beyond the person's control, such as depletion of financial resources or closure of the bar, terminate the drinking rather than the person himself. Persons with loss of control may tend to deny this problem because of its close association with alcohol.

6. Have you ever attended a meeting of Alcoholics Anonymous?

10. Have you ever gone to anyone for help about your drinking?

Questions 6 and 10 inquire about whether the person has sought help for drinking problems.

SHORT MICHIGAN ALCOHOLISM SCREENING TEST*

1. Do you feel you are a normal drinker? (By normal we mean you drink less than or as much as most other people.) (No)[a]
2. Does your wife, husband, a parent, or other near relative ever worry or complain about your drinking? (Yes)
3. Do you ever feel guilty about your drinking? (Yes)
4. Do friends or relatives think you are a normal drinker? (No)
5. Are you able to stop drinking when you want to? (No)
6. Have you ever attended a meeting of Alcoholics Anonymous? (Yes)
7. Has drinking ever created problems between you and your wife, husband, a parent, or other near relative? (Yes)
8. Have you ever gotten into trouble at work because of drinking? (Yes)
9. Have you ever neglected your obligations, your family, or your work for two or more days in a row because you were drinking? (Yes)
10. Have you ever gone to anyone for help about your drinking? (Yes)
11. Have you ever been in a hospital because of drinking? (Yes)
12. Have you ever been arrested for drunken driving, driving while intoxicated, or driving under the influence of alcoholic beverages? (Yes)
13. Have you ever been arrested, even for a few hours, because of other drunken behavior? (Yes)

[a]Alcoholism-indicating responses in parentheses.

Scoring: 0-1 points—nonalcoholic
2 points—possible alcoholic
3 points—alcoholic

---

*Reprinted by permission from Journal of Studies on Alcohol 36:117-126, 1975. Copyright by Journal of Studies on Alcohol, Inc., New Brunswick, N.J. 08903.

8. Have you ever gotten into trouble at work because of drinking?
9. Have you ever neglected your obligations, your family, or your work for two or more days in a row because you were drinking?

Questions 8 and 9 look for impairments on the job or in fulfilling other duties as a result of drinking.

11. Have you ever been in a hospital because of your drinking?

Question 11 examines for evidence of problems with physical health resulting from drinking.

12. Have you ever been arrested for drunken driving, driving while intoxicated, or driving under the influence of alcoholic beverages?
13. Have you ever been arrested, even for a few hours, because of other drunken behavior?

Common types of legal difficulties in alcoholic people are inquired about in questions 12 and 13.

The scoring method for the SMAST is one where each alcoholism-indicating response is given one point. Subjects scoring 0 or 1 point on the SMAST are considered nonalcoholic, those with 2 points possibly alcoholic, and those with 3 points or more alcoholic.[15] Special consideration needs to be given to the person who answers "Yes" to question 6, "Have you ever attended a meeting of Alcoholics Anonymous?" since it is possible for any interested person to attend an open meeting of AA, where the general public is included. It should be remembered, too, that alcoholism-indicating responses pertaining exclusively to the past do not necessarily indicate current alcohol problems.

The SMAST can be a helpful tool in identifying alcoholism by providing objective evidence of its existence. It typically requires only a few minutes to

---

THE CAGE QUESTIONNAIRE*

1. Have you ever felt you should Cut down on your drinking?
2. Have people Annoyed you by criticizing your drinking?
3. Have you ever felt bad or Guilty about your drinking?
4. Have you ever had a drink first thing in the morning to steady your nerves or get rid of a hang-over (Eye-opener)?

Scoring: 2 or 3 out of 4 answered "yes" strongly suggests alcoholism.

---

*From Mayfield D., et al.: The American Journal of Psychiatry 131:1121, 1974. Copyright 1974, the American Psychiatric Association. Reprinted by permission.

administer. It is considered to be a reliable and valid instrument that can be easily incorporated into an existing health assessment form.

A simpler tool designed to diagnose alcoholism is the CAGE Questionnaire (p. 101).[12]

It has been tested for validity among a number of populations of possible alcoholics. It comprises four valuable questions that focus on the main idea of *cutting down* alcohol consumption, *annoyance* by criticism, *guilty* feelings associated with alcohol use, and *"eye openers,"* or early-morning drinking. The title of the questionnaire was derived by extracting the first letter of the four main ideas and formulating the word CAGE. CAGE questions must be asked of the client by the nurse or other worker. In scoring, two or three out of four questions answered "Yes" strongly suggests alcoholism.

RESPONSES TO SCREENING QUESTIONS

The specific tool used to screen for alcoholism, although important, is probably less important than the client's style and quality of response to the questions asked. It is essential to pay close attention to the way in which the person reacts to the questions. Clients can be placed into general categories, according to their initial responses to questions about alcohol use.

The first group, representing the *great majority of people* seen in health care facilities, comprise those who answer the questions *matter-of-factly*. These people are not threatened by questions about alcohol use and show no evidence of any difficulties with alcohol. For this group alcoholism may be ruled out with a reasonable degree of safety unless there are independent indications, such as suspicious physical findings or a spouse's report.[20]

People in the second group also give *reasonably straightforward responses* but *express some concern* about their drinking and, with encouragement, *freely describe the difficulties causing the concern*. This group is composed of *probable early-stage* alcoholic people, including drinkers who use alcohol to relieve symptoms such as insomnia or minor aches and pains, as well as other high-risk individuals, such as a person who has an alcoholic parent. They are gratifying people to work with in that they often respond to intervention as cooperatively as a client with any other developing health problem. It is well to discuss with them, along with a close family member, the symptoms and progressive nature of alcoholism, the desirability of abstaining from alcohol, and if drinking is to continue, the necessity of following a pattern of extreme moderation to avoid serious problems. Throughout subsequent health care visits it is necessary to closely monitor the person's drinking for any evidence or progression toward overt alcoholism.[20]

The third group is characterized by responses that appear to have the goal of *persuading the interviewer there is no alcohol problem*, that the person is simply a social drinker. This group consists of probable *middle-stage alco-*

holic people, whose responses are likely to reflect the elaborate system of rationalizations and denial generated to shield themselves from perceiving reality. In their attempts to defend against revealing any problem with alcohol, people in this group may respond rapidly to questions about alcohol as though they have practiced a response. Or they provide slow, prolonged answers being very careful about what to say. These are the people to whom it is essential to be most carefully attuned so that a more definitive diagnostic assessment may follow.[20]

An additional group consists of *late-stage alcoholic people* who have been in and out of health facilities for many years because of alcoholism. Their lives often revolve around alcohol. When questioned about its use, they readily admit to problems, sometimes with a sad, defeated affect. Some of these people may be severely depressed and suicidal because the cycle of events surrounding alcohol use seems so futile and hopeless to them. Appraising suicidal risk is essential in such instances. A definitive book about suicidology, helpful in accomplishing such appraisal, is available.[6]

A final group includes *people recovering from alcoholism,* sober for varying periods of time, who are *willing and able to talk nondefensively* about their alcoholism. When given the opportunity they can be *potent resources in providing the nurse with useful, firsthand information* about their own experience with alcoholism and sobriety.

CLUES TO ALCOHOLISM

In addition to direct inquiry, the nurse needs to be alert to physical and behavioral clues in clients that may indicate the presence of alcohol-related problems. The clues mentioned in Table 3 are predominantly those manifestations which can be observed by the naked eye or listened for in communication and are not considered exhaustive. One of the most comprehensive compilations of alcoholism symptomatology was formulated through the auspices of the National Council on Alcoholism and is titled *Criteria for the Diagnosis of Alcoholism,* described in Chapter 2.[2] Other references delineating clues indicating alcoholism are also available.[8,16,19]

In practice the nurse combines an understanding of theory, interviewing skills, and the use of her senses, with a knowledge of clues. A nurse provided the following example of how she integrated knowledge and skill with a client:

I stopped at the bedside of a young woman admitted the night before because she had attempted suicide by means of an overdose of tranquilizers. She was seated on her bed wearing short cutoff jeans exposing her legs. Both of her legs were covered with a number of bruises of different ages. As we talked I eventually inquired about the bruises, asking how she had received such a large number. Her response to my question came very rapidly. "I can tell you how I got every single one." She proceeded to explain several of the bruises with an air of confidence and then suddenly burst into tears proclaiming "I drink too much wine and I'm constantly bumping into things." As a result of her admission and the exchange that followed, this woman was transferred from the psychiatric unit where I first contacted her to an alcoholism treatment center where she made excellent progress in learning to manage her alcohol problem.

Table 3. Clues in the appraisal of alcohol-related problems

Physical clues	Behavioral clues
An illness, under treatment, not responding as it should because person may be drinking and not taking medicine as prescribed	Rapid response to questions
"Hash marks" of various ages, particularly in women, on forearms from oven burns	OR
	Very slow prolonged responses to questions about alcohol as though person is being extremely careful about what to say
OR	Preoccupation with alcohol in conversation, with frequent references to being "bombed" or "stoned"
Multiple small cigarette burns on hands or chest, the latter from smoking while drinking in reclining position	Expressing undue concern about welfare of health care provider: "I don't want to bother you, you're busy, just phone in my prescription to drug store"
OR	"Doctor shopping," to get what is wanted, particularly sedative drug prescriptions
Bruises, old and new, particularly at coffee and kitchen table height, due to psychomotor incoordination during intoxication	Coming to scheduled appointment with alcohol on breath
Periorbital and pretibial edema due to retention of fluid following a drunk	Failure to report for health care after an injury for a period of time, as result of not wanting to be seen intoxicated or from fact that pain is masked by anesthetic property of alcohol
Healed or unhealed slash marks across wrists, reflecting high rate of suicide attempts in alcoholic persons	Frequent Monday A.M. absences from work because of "flu"
Flushed face due to vasodilation effects of alcohol	Pattern of taking maximal sick leave during year
Numerous scars on hands and face from falling when drunk or from fights	Frequent calls to health care personnel seeking justification for sick leave
Appearing older than stated age due to debilitating effects of excessive alcohol use	Not performing as well as usual on job
Aseptic necrosis of head of femur without trauma	Poor self-image
Skin stigmata of cirrhosis	Dropping out of nondrinking relationships
Cardiac arrhythmias	Giving up old pastimes and hobbies to spend time drinking
Palpably enlarged liver	Employment choices that facilitate drinking, such as those where a person can function without direct supervision or those which allow business conducted over three-martini luncheon

HIGH-RISK GROUPS

A final dimension to consider in appraising for the presence of possible alcoholism involves the identification of persons who are at a high risk for the development of alcoholism. Epidemiologic and sociologic studies show that a number of factors indicate high risk although there is not complete agreement on the extent of risk for each factor.[2] Such factors include (1) a family history of alcoholism; (2) family history of teetotalism with strong moral prohibitions against alcohol consumption, particularly when the social environment of the person has changed to include drinking; (3) a history of alcoholism or teetotalism in the spouse or family of the spouse; (4) a broken home with marital discord, especially where the father was absent or rejecting but not punitive; (5) the last or almost youngest child in a family; (6) being Irish or Scandinavian in contrast to being Jewish, Chinese, or Italian, the latter reporting a lower incidence of alcoholism than the former cultural groups; (7) female relatives of more than one generation who have a high incidence of recurrent depressions; and (8) heavy smoking, since heavy drinking is often associated with heavy smoking although the reverse need not be true.[2] In acquiring appraisal data, all of these factors need to be considered together with a detailed individual history.

GUIDE FOR QUICK APPRAISAL OF WITHDRAWAL AND EMERGENCY CONDITIONS

The person seen in a health care facility in an intoxicated state, the one with alcohol on his breath who enters an emergency room following trauma, for example, or the suspected or known alcoholic person presenting for treatment all need to be *quickly* appraised for the likelihood of onset of withdrawal symptoms, for the presence of possible emergency conditions, or for both. Questions in the Guide for Quick Appraisal of Impending Withdrawal and Emergency Conditions in Intoxicated and/or Alcoholic Persons (p. 106) assist the nurse in making these appraisals. Answers to questions concerning the latest drinking bout, including its length, quantity of alcohol consumed, and time of last drink, tell the nurse whether or not the person is likely to have a withdrawal reaction, how severe it might be, and when it is likely to occur. For example, a person who has been drinking a pint of whiskey daily for 2 to 10 days and then stops is likely to become tremulous 6 to 8 hours following the last drink. If the person has been drinking a fifth of whiskey for 10 days or more, he is likely to develop delirium tremens.[7,22] The person's past reactions to cessation of drinking and his use of drugs other than alcohol also help predict the current probable withdrawal course. For example, if a person has experienced withdrawal seizures in the past, he is likely to have them again. Additionally, the polydrug abuser will no doubt take longer to detoxify and his symptoms of withdrawal may be more severe.

GUIDE FOR QUICK APPRAISAL OF IMPENDING WITHDRAWAL AND EMERGENCY CONDITIONS IN INTOXICATED AND/OR ALCOHOLIC PERSONS

Aspects affecting impending withdrawal

1. When did you have your last drink?
2. When did you start your last drinking bout?
3. What have you been drinking during this last drinking episode?
4. How much alcohol did you consume each day during your last drinking episode?
5. In the past what reactions have you experienced when you stopped drinking?

☐ Tremors   ☐ Seizures

☐ Hear or see things   ☐ Other _____

☐ DT's

6. Have you ever taken Dilantin or any other drug for seizures?
7. What other medication, if any, are you currently taking?

☐ Prescription   ☐ Over-the-counter   ☐ Street drugs

8. Are you allergic to any drugs?

Potential emergency conditions

9. Do you have any chronic health problems?

☐ Diabetes   ☐ Stomach

☐ Lung   ☐ Liver

☐ Heart   ☐ Other _____

10. Have you recently experienced any of the following?

☐ Pain   ☐ Difficulty keeping your balance

☐ Bleeding   ☐ Double vision

☐ Breathing problems   ☐ Periods of confusion

☐ Vomiting   ☐ Other _____

☐ Diarrhea

11. Have you recently been injured?

☐ In fights   ☐ Fall

☐ Auto crash   ☐ Other _____

Chronic health problems are debilitating and may complicate the course of withdrawal, so questions are asked to determine their presence. Diseases such as diabetes, bronchiectasis, or duodenal ulcer, often neglected during an excessive drinking bout, may need immediate attention concurrent with intervention for withdrawal symptoms. Other conditions in the alcoholic person that may require emergency treatment include hematemesis and double vision (See Chapter 3, Mallory-Weiss, Boerhaave, and Wernicke-Korsakoff syndromes). Finally, questioning the patient about recent injuries as well as examining for evidence of trauma are essential to further determine the presence of conditions requiring immediate intervention.

INTERVIEW GUIDE FOR DETAILED NURSING HISTORY

An interview guide useful in obtaining a *comprehensive* nursing history from persons in early or middle stages of alcoholism or from the chronic alcoholic person who has completed withdrawal or the dry-out period follows (pp. 108 to 115). This guide is *purposefully extensive and thorough* in its coverage. The nurse needs to be familiar with its content and select questions that are appropriate for individual clients rather than expecting to use it in its entirety with every suspected or known alcoholic person. For example, if, after brief screening, it is *suspected* that a client with bleeding gastric ulcers has a drinking problem, the next step in appraisal would be to select and ask further questions from at least those areas of the guide entitled Drinking History and Health History Related To Body Systems: gastrointestinal system. If, on the other hand, the client *acknowledges* alcoholism as a primary health problem, using the majority or all of the questions in the guide is usually appropriate to accomplish a thorough appraisal.

Whether information is gathered in a single sitting or on several separate occasions depends on the client's condition. Long interviews are tiring, so it may be necessary to schedule more than one session to complete the data base with debilitated persons. As a rule it requires at least an hour to complete the entire history-taking process.

The guide is organized to reflect areas especially significant to the alcoholic person: his view of current status, family history, general health history, symptoms related to pathology-prone body systems, drug use other than alcohol, and final questions. The flow of the guide is such that initial questions allow the nurse to become acquainted with the patient regarding family background and present psychosocial status before asking in detail about drinking history. Establishing such a sense of familiarity is especially important with persons who are having difficulty accepting the fact that alcohol may be contributing to their present problems.

The client's responses to questions on the guide will assist the nurse in developing a clear picture of the client's *activities of daily living*, such as patterns of eating and sleeping, as well as the *demands of daily living*, including the client's perception of how adequately he is achieving the expectations he has for himself and the expectations others have for him. The client's *internal resources*, including his physical and psychosocial health status, and the client's *external resources*, such as his home environment, support of family and friends, economic and job status, will also become explicit. It needs to be remembered that the goal of nursing is to determine where

Text continued on p. 115.

DETAILED GUIDE FOR NURSING HISTORY
OF PERSONS WITH ALCOHOL PROBLEMS

GUIDELINES FOR INTERVIEWER

1. Introduce self.
2. Tell interviewee:
   a. Purpose of the interview, including confidentiality of response
   b. Time required to complete interview (approximately 1 hour)
   c. Review of life circumstances may create some discomfort
   d. Refusal to answer specific question(s) is acceptable
3. Obtain verbal permission to proceed with interview.
4. Explore, with additional questions, when responses indicate that more information is needed.

DEMOGRAPHIC DATA

Place of interview _____ Date _____

Name of interviewer _____

Name of interviewee _____ Ethnic group _____ Age _____ Sex _____

Birthplace _____

Last grade attended _____ Are you a veteran? _____

PERSON'S VIEW OF CURRENT STATUS

1. For what reasons did you come to this agency?
2. What do you most want help with at the present time?

FAMILY HISTORY

3. What is your marital status? (Describe your relationship with your spouse.)
4. Do you have children? (Describe your relationship with your children.)
5. How many brothers and sisters do you have?
6. While growing up, were you separated from either parent for any reason? (e.g., death, divorce, running away from home)
7. What did you learn about alcohol when you were growing up? (e.g., from parents, peers)
8. Was alcohol used in your family when you were growing up? If so, what was the pattern of use?
9. Does (or did) anyone in your family have alcohol problems?
10. Does (or did) anyone in your family use drugs other than alcohol excessively?
11. What major illnesses were (are) present in your family?

DETAILED GUIDE FOR NURSING HISTORY
OF PERSONS WITH ALCOHOL PROBLEMS—cont'd

PSYCHOSOCIAL HISTORY

12. Describe your present living arrangement.
    a. With whom do you live?
    b. Does (do) this (these) person(s) use alcohol regularly?
    c. What type of residence do you live in? (e.g., house, apartment, room)
    d. What is the availability and type of transportation that you use?
13. Does your present living arrangement differ greatly from the way you have lived in the past?
14. To whom do you feel close?
15. Does (do) this (these) person(s) use alcohol regularly?
16. What is your occupation?
    a. Do you have special job skills?
    b. Are you presently employed?
    c. If yes, how does this period of treatment affect your employment?
    d. If no, what is your current source of income?
17. If retired, how are you managing this period of your life?
18. Are you actively affiliated with a religious group?
19. What other active affiliations do you have?
20. How do you spend leisure time? (e.g., travel, vacation, activities)
21. What hobbies or special interests do you have?
22. How often and to what degree have you experienced any of the following?
    a. Depression _____
    b. Nervousness (anxiety) _____
    c. Extreme frustration or anger _____
    d. Extreme alienation from others _____
    e. Loneliness _____
    f. Suicidal attempt _____
    g. Other emotional problems _____
23. What do you do when you have these experiences?
24. Have you ever received treatment for emotional problems?

Date	Place
_____	_____
_____	_____
_____	_____

Continued.

DETAILED GUIDE FOR NURSING HISTORY
OF PERSONS WITH ALCOHOL PROBLEMS—cont'd

25. Are you currently taking medication for emotional problems?
26. In general, how do you feel about yourself?
    a. To what extent do you live up to expectations you have for yourself?
    b. How successful are you in meeting expectations of others, including persons such as your spouse, children, employer, and close friends?

DRINKING HISTORY

27. How old were you when you started drinking alcohol?
28. When did you start drinking regularly?
29. How long have you had problems with alcohol?
30. Describe your pattern of drinking?
    a. Frequency? (e.g., daily, weekend, binge)
    b. Kind and amount?
    c. With whom? (e.g., alone, family, friends)
    d. Where?
31. What situations tend to initiate your drinking?
32. When are you most likely to drink heavily?
33. When did you have your last drink?
34. When did you start your last drinking bout?
35. What have you been drinking during this last drinking episode?
36. How much alcohol did you consume each day during your last drinking episode?
37. Has your drinking created problems for you in any of the following areas?
    ☐ Spouse   ☐ Children
    ☐ Family   ☐ School
    ☐ Friends   ☐ Other _____
    ☐ Job
38. Have you ever been injured because of drinking?
    ☐ In fights   ☐ Falls
    ☐ Auto crashes   ☐ Other _____
39. Have you ever been arrested because of drinking?
    ☐ Driving while intoxicated   ☐ Fights
    ☐ Drunk in public   ☐ Other _____
40. Have you ever been in prison or jail because of drinking?
41a. How have you managed any of the above problems when they have occurred?

DETAILED GUIDE FOR NURSING HISTORY
OF PERSONS WITH ALCOHOL PROBLEMS—cont'd

DRINKING HISTORY—cont'd

41b. What previous treatments have you had for alcohol problems?

Date

Place

_____ _____

_____ _____

_____ _____

42. When not drinking, do you experience craving?
    a. Are you experiencing craving now?
    b. How have you dealt with craving in the past? .
43. When you are drinking heavily, how do you spend a typical day?

GENERAL HEALTH HISTORY

44. Describe your current state of health.
45. What major illnesses or hospitalizations have you had that you have not already mentioned?

HEALTH HISTORY RELATED TO BODY SYSTEMS
Gastrointestinal system

46. What is your usual eating pattern?
    a. When not drinking?
    b. When drinking?
47. Are you on a special diet?
48. What kinds and amounts of beverages do you drink per day other than alcohol?

    Regular coffee _____ Decaffeinated coffee _____ Tea _____
    Water _____ Soft drinks _____ Juices _____ Milk _____
49. Do you experience any of the following?
    ☐ Irritation of mouth, tongue,   ☐ Abdominal pain
      and/or throat   ☐ Nausea
    ☐ Stomach pain   ☐ Constipation
    ☐ Heartburn or gas   ☐ Other _____
    ☐ Vomiting or dry heaves
    ☐ Diarrhea
50. Have you ever vomited blood? If yes, when?
51. Have you ever had stomach ulcers or other stomach problems?
52. How frequently and for what reason do you use aspirin?

Continued.

DETAILED GUIDE FOR NURSING HISTORY
OF PERSONS WITH ALCOHOL PROBLEMS—cont'd

Gastrointestinal system—cont'd

53. What medications do you use to relieve stomach distress?
54. Do you have hemorrhoids?
55. Have you had bleeding from your bowels?
56. Have you noted a change in the color of your stool?
   ☐ Clay colored   ☐ Black   ☐ Bright red
57. What medications do you use to relieve abdominal or bowel distress?
58. Have you ever been told you have problems with your pancreas?
59. Have you ever had jaundice?
60. Have you ever been told you have problems with your liver?
61. Do you have diabetes? If yes, what medication do you take?

Neurologic system

62. What changes, if any, have you noticed as to the amount of alcohol it takes to bring about the effects you desire?
63. What reactions do you experience when you stop drinking?
   ☐ Tremors   ☐ DT's
   ☐ Seizures   ☐ Other _____
   ☐ Hear or see things
64. Have you ever taken Dilantin or any other drug for seizures?
65. Have you ever been unable to remember later what occurred while you were drinking?
66. Do you experience any of the following?
   ☐ Tingling, pain, or numbness in hands or feet
   ☐ Muscle pain in legs or arms
   ☐ Difficulty in keeping your balance
   ☐ Double vision
   ☐ Periods of mental confusion
67. Describe any problems you experience with your sleep?
   a. Do you feel rested after a night's sleep?
   b. What do you do when you are unable to sleep?

Cardiovascular and respiratory system

68. Do you experience any of the following?
   ☐ Swelling of the hands and feet   ☐ Chest pain
   ☐ Shortness of breath   ☐ Irregular heartbeats
   ☐ Rapid heartbeat   ☐ Other _____
   ☐ Varicose veins

DETAILED GUIDE FOR NURSING HISTORY
OF PERSONS WITH ALCOHOL PROBLEMS—cont'd

Cardiovascular and respiratory system—cont'd

69. Have you ever been told you have any of the following?
    - ☐ High blood pressure
    - ☐ Anemias of any type
    - ☐ Any other blood disorder
70. What, if any, medication are you taking for heart disease?
71. Do you experience any of the following?
    - ☐ Frequent colds
    - ☐ Tuberculosis
    - ☐ Coughing up blood
    - ☐ Pneumonia
    - ☐ Chronic cough
    - ☐ Coughing excessive amounts of phlegm
    - ☐ Other _____
72. Do you smoke?
    - a. If yes, how many packs a day?
    - b. If no, have you ever smoked?

Musculoskeletal system

73. Do you experience any of the following?
    - ☐ Frequent fractures
    - ☐ Muscle swelling
    - ☐ Muscle pain or tenderness
    - ☐ Muscle weakness

Integument

74. Do you experience any of the following?
    - ☐ Sores that heal poorly
    - ☐ Wine sores
    - ☐ Dermatitis
    - ☐ Hair loss
    - ☐ Frequent boils
    - ☐ Psoriasis
    - ☐ Small bright spots on skin (petechiae)
    - ☐ Reddened palms
75. Do you bruise easily?

Genitourinary system

76. Do you experience any of the following?
    - ☐ Painful urination
    - ☐ Blood in the urine
    - ☐ Frequency of urination
    - ☐ Difficulty in passing urine
77. Women:
    - a. Are you sexually active?
    - b. Are you able to receive satisfaction from your sexual encounters?
    - c. What method of contraception do you use?
    - d. Describe any changes in your sex life since you have been drinking heavily.

Continued.

DETAILED GUIDE FOR NURSING HISTORY
OF PERSONS WITH ALCOHOL PROBLEMS—cont'd

Genitourinary system—cont'd

    e. Are your menstrual periods regular?

    f. Do you experience a buildup of tension prior to your period?

    g. Have your periods changed since you began drinking heavily?

    h. Have you ever been pregnant?

        (1) Number of live births?

        (2) Number of abortions?

        (3) Have you given birth to an infant with defects?

        (4) Are you pregnant now?

78. Men:

    a. Are you sexually active?

    b. Are you able to receive satisfaction from your sexual encounters?

    c. What method of contraception do you use?

    d. Describe any changes in your sex life since you have been drinking heavily.

DRUG TAKING OTHER THAN ALCOHOL

79. What drugs do you take that you haven't mentioned?

    □ Prescribed drugs _____

    □ Over-the-counter drugs _____

    □ Drugs obtained on the street _____

80. How do you administer the drugs? (e.g., mainlining [intravenous], skin popping [subcutaneous])

81. What is your usual manner of taking drugs?

    □ As directed   □ Less than directed

    □ More than directed   □ According to what you feel you need

82. Have you experienced any of the following as a result of your use of street drugs?

    □ Gum infections   □ Blood poisoning

    □ Infections at site of injection   □ Hepatitis

    □ Abscesses   □ Drug overdose

83. Are you allergic to any drugs?

FINAL QUESTIONS

84. What are your ideas for managing your drinking when you leave this agency?

85. Are there any further comments you would like to make?

86. Are there any questions you would like to ask?

DETAILED GUIDE FOR NURSING HISTORY
OF PERSONS WITH ALCOHOL PROBLEMS—cont'd

GUIDELINES FOR USE OF THE DATA

Describe your overall observations of the client, including mood, attitude, intelligence, ability to relate, social skills, general physical and emotional health, level of orientation, reliability of information given.

Based on the appraisal data, determine the client's activities and demands of daily living and his external and internal resources.

Identify and describe existing imbalances between the client's daily living requirements and his resources for meeting these requirements.

Formulate nursing diagnoses for the imbalances.

Prescribe nursing management strategies appropriate for correcting the imbalances.

Depending on the client's health status, discuss the strategies with him to determine their acceptability and relevance to his life-style.

Rework management strategies, taking client's suggestions into consideration.

---

imbalances exist for the client in any of the four components, activities and demands of daily living and internal and external resources, so that nursing diagnosis and management strategies may be developed.

The nursing history tool is only a guide. When positive findings are identified, the nurse needs to formulate, on the spot, additional appropriate questions to clarify symptomatology. For example, when the person answers affirmatively that alcohol use has caused involvement in fights, questions need to be asked about matters such as frequency and extent of injury. It is always important for the nurse to ask additional questions to clarify how alcohol use interferes with the person's fulfilling the activities and demands of daily living and to formulate questions to explicate internal and external resources for coping with life.

As stated, questions on the guide are organized into specific content areas. To clarify the rationale on which the guide is based, overall purposes of questions in each content area will be highlighted.

Person's view of current status

The first questions are intended to permit the person to state his reason for seeking help and to name what help is desired at the present time. With these questions the client is expected to give a review of his current troubles as he sees them. Allowing the person to be spontaneous during this account, with minimal verbal prompting from the nurse, is useful in gaining a picture of the client's view of himself. The flow of words from the client at this point may sound somewhat disorganized and contain an intermingling of facts and feelings. Clarification can be postponed in favor of encouraging spontaneous expression. The nurse's task in this portion of the interview is to listen carefully, make mental or written notes of questions to ask later, refocus the communication if the client strays too far from the subject, and terminate remarks when further elaboration would be redundant or unnecessary. In the sets of questions that follow, the nurse takes the lead and poses specific questions, expecting to obtain a clear understanding of the person's main difficulties.

Family history

To comprehend the environment in which the client's disturbances with alcohol occurred, questions on family background are asked. Identifying parental attitudes and behaviors regarding alcohol may help clarify some of the conflicts the person currently suffers. Does the client's present use of alcohol deviate greatly from parental behavior, or is it similar to that displayed by family members? Typically, a familial background of alcoholism occurs with great frequency in the lives of persons who themselves develop alcoholism.[4] Establishing this connection, if indeed it is present, can be helpful in diminishing the person's guilt about his present illness. Also it can be used to set expectations regarding the responsibility of alcoholic parents to inform their offspring about the familial nature of alcoholism. When parents assume this responsibility, the likelihood of succeeding generations making informed choices about alcohol use will undoubtedly increase.

Psychosocial history

Alcoholism almost always interferes significantly with the person's psychologic and social status. Excessive drinking ultimately replaces interpersonal relationships as a source of gratification, and many chronic alcoholic people are totally bereft of meaningful friendships and family ties. A number of clients have answered the question, "To whom do you feel close?" with the simple statement, "My bottle." The most difficult person in the world to become rehabilitated is the lone alcoholic, the one with no spouse or family and with few other external resources. Patients who have intact emotional ties are more likely to respond favorably to treatment. Identifying the client's support system in the appraisal process and taking steps later to reestablish deteriorating links may be a key aspect to recovery.

Other external resources affecting outcome of alcoholism include job status and the person's ability to use time in ways other than drinking. If alcohol is to be removed from person's life, the next logical question is, "What is to take its place?" Does the person have nondrinking affiliations or hobbies to draw upon, or is there a need to establish new associations and outlets?

Depression and suicide figure prominently in the lives of people who drink excessively. Alcohol, pharmacologically, is a central nervous system depressant and, when drunk to excess, can, itself produce depressive feelings. Elimination of large quantities of alcohol from a person's life promotes relief of sad feelings. Other people who experience serious depressive episodes may learn to self-medicate with alcohol to dull intensely felt emotional pain to the extent of developing alcoholism. The combination of serious depression and alcoholism greatly increases the likelihood of suicidal behavior. Compared with the general population, alcoholic persons more frequently attempt and complete suicide.[1] In appraising alcoholic persons who feel sad and hopeless, it is necessary to determine if a depressive disorder underlies the alcoholism. If so, treatment for both the alcoholism and the depression will need to be instituted.

Determining if the person is currently taking medication for emotional problems is important in subsequent management. The alcoholic client who has been taking chlordiazepoxide (Librium) or diazepam (Valium), for example, is likely to experience more severe withdrawal symptoms because of the augmentation of alcohol in the presence of a minor tranquilizer.

Drinking history

Information about the patient's drinking history is essential for a variety of reasons. Dangerous patterns of drinking can be unveiled through answers to questions such as the frequency and amount of alcohol intake. Patterns of drinking that have been identified as potentially dangerous are drinking enough to be moderately high several times a week, drinking enough to get really drunk once a week, and drinking to oblivion (spree drinking) once a month.[18] There are other patterns of drinking that may be equally harmful, and not every person who exhibits these behaviors is alcoholic. What is meant by the patterns is that the person who exhibits them runs a much higher risk of developing problem drinking or alcoholism. Identifying such a person long before the advanced symptoms of alcoholism are entrenched allows the nurse to initiate primary prevention strategies, such as providing information, wirtten and verbal, about alcohol and alcoholism. Questions about the latest drinking bout help the nurse determine whether the client is likely to have a withdrawal reaction, how severe it might be, and when it might occur as described earlier in this chapter (p. 105).

Identifying the gamut of problems resulting from drinking helps the nurse assess the degree and manner in which alcohol has encroached on the person's daily life. What problems, if any, has alcohol use created with family members or on the job? Has the person experienced injuries or legal entanglements as a result of drinking?

Craving, defined variously as an "irresistible desire" or "overpowering need" for alcohol, is a phenomenon common to many alcoholic people about which little is known.[11] One reason why alcoholic persons may fail to refrain from use of alcohol is the experience of craving. Increased understanding of craving and its management could lead to a decrease in the incidence of relapse during periods of recovery.

Obtaining specific information about how the person spends a typical day often yields important appraisal data on the activities and demands of daily living. Emphasis needs to be placed on learning about the times during a usual 24-hour period when alcohol use is most likely to ensue, increase, or diminish. Is there a relationship between stress, experienced variously by the person as boredom, loneliness, nervousness, or being overtaxed, and alcohol use? When such connections are identified, measures can be taken to reduce or eliminate the stressor and alternative means of handling the situation can be explored.

It is around the drinking history that the client's denial of a problem with alcohol may be at a peak. The nursing history tool does not screen for denial. Skill in interviewing and close attention to the client's manner in answering drinking history questions can assist the nurse in determining the presence of denial.

General health history

Chronic alcoholic persons have been described as being "museums of pathology," with greatly diminished internal resources. They often have experienced numerous hospitalizations and major illnesses. On the other hand, persons who have been alcoholic for shorter durations may have few, if any, persistent health problems. Questions in this section allow the client to describe how he perceives his present and past general health status. Does the client believe himself to be fit and robust, or rather does he convey feeling weak and frail? Does the nurse's perception match the client's? Some alcoholic persons seem unaware of deteriorating health, possibly because of the dulling effect of alcohol on the drinker's discernment of physical and emotional ills.

Health history related to body systems

Although almost every organ of the body is finally affected by alcohol, certain body systems are more susceptible to damage than others. Questions in this section are aimed at eliciting the client's unique and specific health problems within different body systems and determining how he is coping with them. Most of these problems and their symptoms have been described in Chapter 3 and will be summarized here. These data are of special importance to the nurse in determining the client's internal resources, especially those involving endurance and physical health.

The section begins with questions related to the injurious effects of alcohol on the gastrointestinal tract, including the client's experience with symptoms such as stomach distress or diarrhea. Questions about diet are important because persons who drink large quantities of alcohol simultaneously have high caloric intakes and tend not to feel hungry. Alcohol replaces nutritious foods, leading to malnutrition. Even alcoholic persons with adequate food intake experience malnutrition due to malabsorption of carbohydrates, amino acids, vitamins, and iron.[10]

Liver disease is a commonly recognized consequence of heavy drinking, and clients often raise questions about the condition of their liver during appraisal interviews. Although liver disease may be diagnosed readily by physical examination or laboratory tests, the person may not be aware of having liver dysfunction unless symptoms are acute or well advanced.

Acute and chronic pancreatitis are common in alcoholic persons, causing severe abdominal pain and digestive disturbance. Pancreatitis tends to recur as heavy drinking continues. People who have had pancreatitis usually have vivid memories of the episode.

Alcohol in any amount affects the central nervous system. Acute intoxication, alcohol dependence, peripheral neuropathy, and the Wernicke-Korsakoff syndrome are examples of the effect of alcohol on nerve cells. Tolerance results, too, from the altered sensitivity of nerve cells to alcohol. If tolerance is well established, it can be assumed the person is no stranger to alcohol. When a person describes having "lost" the ability to handle large amounts of alcohol, tolerance is diminishing. This usually indicates an advanced stage of alcoholism.

Questions about past reactions to withdrawal from alcohol are important in anticipating current responses. If a person has had withdrawal seizures on a prior occasion, he is likely to experience them again. Giving appropriate medication promptly to prevent seizures is indicated.

Sleep disturbances are prominent in alcoholic persons, with interference in the ability to fall asleep and to have a deep, restful sleep. Often the alcoholic person uses alcohol as a sedative in a futile attempt to counteract sleep disturbances initially caused by excessive alcohol intake, only perpetuating the drinking-insomnia cycle. Learning alternative methods of promoting sleep is an obvious need of such a person.

Diseases of the cardiovascular system, too, are related to alcohol consumption. The clinical findings of alcoholic cardiomyopathy are the same as cardiac failure from any cause, and obtaining an accurate drinking history is the means whereby etiology is differentiated.

Table 4. Some drug interactions with alcohol*

Drug	Effect	Probable mechanism
Antabuse (disulfiram)	Flushing, diaphoresis, hyperventilation, vomiting, confusion, drowsiness	Inhibits intermediary metabolism of alcohol
Anticoagulants, oral	Increased anticoagulant effect with acute intoxication	Reduced metabolism
	Decreased anticoagulant effect after chronic alcohol abuse	Enhanced microsomal enzyme activity
Antihistamines	Increased CNS depression	Additive
Antimicrobials		
Chloramphenicol (Chloromycetin; and others)	Minor Antabuse-like reaction	Inhibits intermediary metabolism of alcohol
Furazolidone (Furoxone)	Minor Antabuse-like reaction	Inhibits intermediary metabolism of alcohol
Griseofulvin (Fulvicin-U/F; and others)	Minor Antabuse-like reaction	Inhibits intermediary metabolism of alcohol
Isoniazid (many mfrs.)	Decreased effect after chronic alcohol abuse	Undetermined
Metronidazole (Flagyl)	Minor Antabuse-like reaction	Possible CNS effect
Quinacrine (Atabrine)	Minor Antabuse-like reaction	Inhibits intermediary metabolism of alcohol
Hypoglycemics		
Chlorpropamide (Diabinese)	Minor Antabuse-like reaction	Inhibits intermediary metabolism of alcohol
Phenformin (DBI; Meltrol)	Lactic acidosis	Additive
Tolbutamide (Orinase)	Decreased hypoglycemic effect after chronic alcohol abuse	Enhanced microsomal enzyme activity
	Increased hypoglycemic effect with ingestion of alcohol, particularly in fasting patients	Suppression of gluconeogenesis

*From The Medical Letter **19:**48 (Issue 471), Jan. 28, 1977, 56 Harrison St., New Rochelle, N.Y. 10801. Reprinted with permission.

Table 4. Some drug interactions with alcohol—cont'd

Drug	Effect	Probable mechanism
Tolbutamide (Orinase)—cont'd	Minor Antabuse-like reaction	Inhibits intermediary metabolism of alcohol
Narcotics	Increased CNS depression with acute intoxication	Additive
Salicylates	Gastrointestinal bleeding	Additive
Sedatives and tranquiliziers		
Barbiturates	Increased CNS depression with acute intoxication	Additive; reduced metabolism
	Decreased sedative effect after chronic alcohol abuse	Enhanced microsomal enzyme activity; decreased CNS sensitivity
Chloral hydrate (Noctec; and others)	Prolonged hypnotic effect	Mutual potentiation
Chlordiazepoxide (Librium; and others)	Increased CNS depression	Additive
Chlorpromazine (Thorazine; Chlor-PZ)	Increased CNS depression	Additive; inhibits oxidation of alcohol
Clorazepate (Azene; Tranxene)	Increased CNS depression	Additive
Diazepam (Valium)	Increased CNS depression	Additive; possible increased absorption
Meprobamate (Miltown; and others)	Increased CNS depression with acute intoxication	Additive; reduced metabolism
	Decreased sedative effect after chronic alcohol abuse	Enhanced microsomal enzyme activity
Oxazepam (Serax)	Increased CNS depression	Additive
Others†		
Phentolamine (Regitine)	Minor Antabuse-like reaction	Inhibits intermediary metabolism of alcohol
Phenytoin (Dilantin; and others)	Increased anticonvulsant effect with acute intoxication	Reduced metabolism
	Decreased anticonvulsant effect after chronic alcohol abuse	Enhanced microsomal enzyme activity

†Many alcoholic beverages contain tyramine, which can cause reactions with MAO inhibitors (Medical Letter **19:5,** 1977).

Blood pressure and pulse are typically elevated during alcohol withdrawal so that careful monitoring of vital signs needs to be instituted both during and after withdrawal phases. This is important for the diagnosis of cardiac conditions as well as for essential hypertension.

Alcoholic persons are in jeopardy for respiratory disease, including chronic bronchitis, bronchiectasis, pneumonia, lung abscess, aspiration pneumonia, and tuberculosis. It is rare to find an alcoholic person who does not smoke heavily, adding to the likelihood of respiratory difficulties.

Alcoholic persons have a propensity for trauma. Many have sustained numerous fractures and bruises during bouts of intoxication. A lesser known malady often overlooked or dismissed in the alcoholic person is muscle involvement, including symptoms of both acute and chronic alcoholic myopathy.

Alcoholic persons have increased liability to infections in general and a greater mortality when infected. The inhibition of leukocyte migration into areas of inflammation induced by small amounts of alcohol probably plays an important part in the poor resistance of alcoholic people to bacterial infections.[9] Questions about bladder functioning may elicit responses about difficulties associated with infection or other disorders of the urinary tract. Persons who drink excessively experience diuresis as blood alcohol levels are rising, and for that reason they may respond affirmatively to the question about frequency of urination.

Alcoholism, as well as other drug dependencies, is usually accompanied by greatly reduced sexual interest and performance.[3] However, the alcoholic person does not, as a rule, associate diminished desire or lowered ability to perform sexually with alcohol intake. Questions about sexuality are aimed at opening discussion about a subject around which misinformation and discomfort often exist for both the nurse and client. The nurse who is inexperienced in assessing a client's sexual history may find additional readings on the subject helpful. One such reference is suggested.[21]

When appraising women with alcohol problems who are sexually active, it is of special importance to address the issue of contraception. These women need to know about the possible effects of drugs such as nicotine, caffeine, and alcohol on the fetus. If an alcoholic woman has already given birth to an infant with fetal alcohol syndrome, her needs for special counseling may be intense and the child may need to be referred to a clinic where thorough appraisal and management can be implemented.

Men, too, need to be queried about the responsibility they are assuming for contraception if they are sexually active. Intoxication often causes people to be careless about the precautions necessary to prevent unwanted pregnancies. Men need to be educated about the potential dangers to offspring when pregnancy, alcohol, and other drug use are combined. It may be necessary to ask men who encourage and expect their spouses to drink with them to cease doing so when the woman is anticipating pregnancy or is pregnant.

The effects of alcoholism on the skin, the largest organ of the body, have not been studied thoroughly, mainly because there are more serious diseases to be expected in internal organs. Although extensive data are lacking, changes of the skin resulting from long-term alcohol use can be expected. Some of these are a result of liver damage; others are due to vascular responses and to changes in blood and blood-forming organs. Changes in the skin alone are not diagnostic of alcoholism. In combination with other symptomatology, skin changes can alert the nurse to the possible presence of alcoholism.

Drug taking other than alcohol

It is uncommon to find persons who abuse only one drug. Most alcoholic people are multidrug abusers, and this is especially true with youth and women. Moreover, a person's pattern of taking drugs is likely to be erratic. Overindulgence may be the practice at one time and complete omission at another. Such a pattern is especially disruptive when a client is being treated for a condition requiring prescription drugs such as antibiotics for a urinary tract infection.

In this section of the guide, appraisal is directed toward determining whether the client is taking prescribed, over-the-counter, or illicitly obtained drugs. Some drugs, in combination with alcohol, can lead to complications because of their synergistic or antagonistic interactions. A listing of some drug interactions with alcohol is found in Table 4; other effects are discussed in additional references.[5, 13] It is essential to inform both alcoholic and nonalcoholic persons about the adverse, sometimes fatal, outcome of combining alcohol with specific drugs, prescribed or not.

Final questions

The final section may yield some of the most useful appraisal data of the entire history-taking process. Learning about what plans, if any, the client has for dealing with his alcohol problem is essential in determining care. Clients who have given this matter little thought will need motivational counseling before much action toward recovery can be anticipated.

REFERENCES

1. Benesohn, H.S., and Resnik, H. I. P.: A jigger of alcohol, a dash of depression, and bitters: a suicidal mix, Annals of the New York Academy of Sciences **233**:40-46, 1974.
2. Criteria Committee, National Council on Alcoholism: Criteria for the diagnosis of alcoholism, Annals of Internal Medicine **77**:249-258, 1972; American Journal of Psychiatry **129**:127-135, 1972.

3. Fort, J.: Sex and drugs, Postgraduate Medicine **58**:133-136, 1975.
4. Goodwin, D.: Is alcoholism hereditary? New York, 1976, Oxford University Press.
5. Hansten, P. D.: Drug interactions, Philadelphia, 1975, Lea & Febiger.
6. Hatton, C. L., Valente, S. M., and Rink, A.: Suicide assessment and intervention, New York, 1977, Appleton-Century-Crofts.
7. Johnson, R. B.: Alcohol withdrawal syndrome, Quarterly Journal of Studies on Alcohol **1** (suppl.):66-76, Nov., 1961.
8. Knott, D. H., Fink, R. D., and Beard, J. D.: Unmasking alcohol abuse, American Family Physician **10**:123-128, 1978.
9. Lindenbaum, J.: Hematologic effects of alcohol In Kissin, B., and Begleiter, H., editors: The biology of alcoholism, Vol. 3, Clinical pathology, New York, 1974, Plenum Press, Inc.
10. Lorber, S. H., Dinoso, V. P., and Chey, W. Y.: Disease of the gastrointestinal tract In Kissin, B., and Begleiter, H., editors: Biology of alcoholism. Vol. 3, Clinical pathology, New York, 1973, Plenum Press, Inc.
11. Ludwig, A. M., and Wikler, A.: Craving and relapse to drink, Quarterly Journal of Studies on Alcohol **35**:108-130, 1974.
12. Mayfield, D., et al.: The CAGE Questionnaire: validation of a new alcoholism screening instrument, American Journal of Psychiatry **131**:1121-1123, 1974.
13. Seixas, F. A.: Alcohol and its drug interactions, Annals of Internal Medicine **83**:86-92, 1975.
14. Seixas, F. A.: The course of alcoholism In Estes, N., and Heinemann, E., editors: Alcoholism, development, consequences and interventions, St. Louis, 1977, The C. V. Mosby Co.
15. Selzer, M. L., Vinokur, A., and van Rooijen, L.: A self-administered Short Michigan Alcoholism Screening Test (SMAST), Journal of Studies on Alcohol **36**:117-126, 1975.
16. Shropshire, R. W.: The hidden face of alcoholism, Geriatrics **30**:99-102, 1975.
17. Some drug interactions with alcohol, The Medical Letter **19**:48, (Issue 471); Jan. 28. 1977.
18. The National Center for Alcohol Education: The community health nurse and alcohol related problems, Rockville, Md., June, 1978, National Institute on Alcohol Abuse and Alcoholism.
19. Round table: Picking up alcoholism in your patient family, Patient Care **8**:40+, Sept. 1, 1974.
20. Weinberg, J.: Interview techniques for diagnosing alcoholism, American Family Physician **9**:107-115, 1974.
21. Whitley, M. P., and Willingham, D.: Adding a sexual assessment to the health interview, Journal of Psychiatric Nursing and Mental Health Services **16**:17-27, April, 1978.
22. Wolfe, S., and Maurice, V.: Physiological basis of the alcohol withdrawal syndrome In Mello, N. K., and Mendelson, J. H., editors: Recent advances in studies of alcoholism, Interdisciplinary Symposium, National Center for Prevention and Control of Alcoholism, Washington, D.C., 1971, U.S. Government Printing Office.

CHAPTER 7

Appraisal by interview

client fears, nurses' attitudes, interview phases

It might be expected that alcoholic persons would want to tell everything that could possibly influence their health in an appraisal interview. The fact is this society does not endorse open discussion of alcoholism and its many related predicaments. For this reason many people will conceal facts of extreme importance to their health, even their lives, because of difficulties in openly acknowledging the presence of alcohol problems. It happens, then, that alcoholism may be purposefully hidden *by* the drinker but at the same time alcoholism is sometimes hidden *from* the drinker. Many people, especially those with early stage alcoholism, do not directly associate internal experiences of various physical symptoms such as insomnia, irritability, and restlessness with their abuse of alcohol until the relationship is made clear to them. In other instances involving external events such as job difficulties or family disruptions, alcohol abuse is not readily identified as a causative agent by the drinker. The widespread acceptance of alcohol as an integral part of society enables people to continue drinking even when difficulties are experienced as a result of its use. Because of these factors, much of the responsibility for diagnosing alcoholism will fall to health care personnel, including the nurse.

What are ingredients of successful interviewing for purposes of acquiring accurate data from alcoholic persons? It is the purpose of this chapter to describe potential interferences in this process, including fears of the alcoholic client and attitudes of the nurse. The phases of obtaining health history data and ways to acquire the data successfully are also described.

FEARS OF CLIENT

For most people, admission of a major problem with alcohol is charged with a great deal of emotion, most notably fear of rejection, fear of incurability, and fear of curability.[1] The *fear of rejection* is associated with the social disapproval and personal feelings of guilt and inadequacy involved in alcoholism. One person expressed his fear of rejection by saying, "Once you admit you're an alcoholic, people aren't going to trust you, they aren't going to have anything to do with you."

A second fear, *fear of incurability,* involves the person's attempt to escape a label that is often associated with inevitable destruction, such as the drinker may have already witnessed in a family member or friend. The last great fear of the alcoholic person is the exact opposite of the fear of incurability, yet often exists simultaneously with it. It is the *fear of recovery.* Facing life free of alcohol can be extremely frightening for the person who relies on it to solve every problem, albeit negatively, no matter how minor. When alcohol is removed, the question that must be faced is, "What will take its place?" Recovering from alcoholism often means adopting a completely new life-style, one that initially is fraught with overwhelming uncertainties about success. Because of these major fears, and probably many others, alcoholic people often become involved in self-deception about their drinking, sometimes to such degrees as to approach delusion.

One of the major differences between interviewing an alcoholic person and someone with another illness is the amount of defensiveness commonly manifested by the alcoholic client.[6] If the nurse will anticipate that defensiveness is part of the symptomatology of alcoholism, she will be in a position to monitor her responses, taking care not to become involved in reciprocal defensiveness. At the same time the nurse will be more willing to make the extra efforts necessary to obtain adequate appraisal data. It makes no more sense to become annoyed with the alcoholic person who minimizes a drinking problem than it does to react with anger to a person with a duodenal ulcer who experiences "heartburn."

NURSES' ATTITUDES

No doubt the most important element in determining the success of the appraisal interview concerns the nurse's attitudes toward alcohol, alcoholism, and alcoholic persons. Most nurses need to scrutinize their feelings on these matters carefully before it is possible to discuss alcohol use effectively with clients. It can also be anticipated that some people experiencing alcohol problems will directly query the nurse about whether she uses alcohol. To respond nondefensively and constructively, the nurse needs to be confident that her use, if it occurs at all, is not self-destructive in any way or harmful to others. The following is a set of questions that the nurse may wish to use in developing a dialogue about drinking with another person or group of people for purposes of generating open and honest thought about alcohol and its meaning in one's personal life.

Do I drink?

    If so, when, where, how much, how often, for what reasons?

    If not, what causes me to abstain?

What did I learn about alcohol when I was growing up?

What are my attitudes now about alcohol?

What do I experience when I see a drunk man? A drunk woman?

Do I look negatively on drunken behavior in others and yet overindulge on occasion myself?

Can I distinguish between social drinking, the use of alcohol in moderation, and heavy drinking?

Can I talk rationally with others about their use of alcohol, especially when their patterns of drinking differ greatly from mine?

What kind of a model am I regarding alcohol use for a younger person who may be emulating my conduct?

In examining one's beliefs about alcohol-related matters, it is not uncommon to uncover at least two attitudinal problems.[6] One is the historic view of alcoholism as a moral problem, which most people still carry deep inside. Such feelings may lead to a subtle communication of hostility or condemnation that will block the success of the interview and of establishing a relationship. The other problem is the tendency to judge the deviance of the client's drinking pattern by comparison with one's own drinking habits. This response is more common when interacting with the alcoholic person whose life still appears intact and similar to that of the nurse. If the nurse drinks little or not at all, she may exaggerate the client's drinking problems, whereas a nurse with heavier alcohol intake may be highly reluctant to identify as alcoholic anyone who apparently drinks less than she does. These tendencies may be altered if the nurse remembers that alcoholism is not a moral problem and if the results of drinking, rather than the amount consumed, are made paramount in the appraisal process. People who repeatedly end up behaving in an objectionable manner after even moderate alcohol intake have alcohol problems, whereas people who drink larger quantities without behavioral or physical sequelae may be problem free.

PHASES OF OBTAINING INTERVIEW DATA

Obtaining the health history data needed for appraisal of the alcoholic person occurs in several phases including (1) the preparatory phase, (2) client interview, and (3) reordering the data.

Preparatory phase

In preparing to acquire appraisal data, the nurse needs to be sensitive to the fact that the information exchanged between herself and the client may be affected by a number of factors. The *personal characteristics of the nurse,* for example, may influence the communication that occurs. When the client is considerably older than the nurse, the client may adopt a parental attitude toward the nurse, sometimes behaving toward her as though she were a daughter. On the other hand, when the nurse is older and the client youthful, the client may relate to the nurse as he does to his mother. Clients of either sex may feel inhibited about discussing certain topics with a nurse of the opposite sex. The dress and overall appearance of the nurse can be influential in the response received from the client. The nurse who wears the traditional uniform, cap, and pin may represent staunch authority or strong protection to some people, and their reaction will be in accordance with their perception, rational or irrational, of persons in positions of power. In contrast, the casually attired nurse will convey quite another set of messages to the client regarding the image of a professional nurse.

In all instances where the nurse is relating directly with the client, it is important *to observe good personal hygiene and to be discreet in the use of cosmetics*. Strongly scented perfumes or after-shave lotions may be highly irritating, for example, to the person with asthma or may only increase the nauseated person's sensation of gastric distress. The nurse's personal *use of colored nail polish needs to be omitted* in the care setting, since it may prohibit her from making observations such as comparing the client's nail bed color with her own. The conscientious nurse will want to take into account these seemingly minor details and make allowances accordingly to attain the overall success of the appraisal process to the greatest possible extent. The goal is to make certain that nothing is done through careless attention to demeanor or appearance to undermine the nurse's status as a competent professional person in the eyes of the client.

A second aspect of the preparatory phase includes *selecting the interview setting*. Determining where the interview will be conducted needs to be done with care, since the success of the exchange may hinge closely on this factor. The setting needs to assure privacy so that both the nurse and the client can communicate with freedom from concerns about being overheard or interrupted. The interview needs to be conducted in a quiet, comfortable, well-lighted place where there is no need to strain to see or hear. Preferably the nurse and client should be seated face to face with enough space between them so that both are comfortable and at ease. The client should be fully visible to the nurse for observation purposes. There should be no barriers such as a desk or bed between them. The nurse's voice tone needs to be adjusted to fit the setting and the client's hearing capacity.

A *system for recording the data* needs to be determined prior to the interview, otherwise valuable information may be forgotten or inaccurately recalled later. The most common method is for the nurse to write in responses to questions on the interview guide as the interview proceeds. When this method is used, the nurse needs to maintain responsiveness to the client, such as through frequent eye contact, and avoid becoming overly engrossed in recording answers in the guide. In some instances, when the client is physically and mentally capable, he may be asked to record responses to the questions. As an alternative to writing responses, the interview can be tape recorded, leaving the participants free to concentrate solely on the exchange as it occurs. If this method is used, it is customary in most settings first to obtain the written permission of the client to make an audio-tape of the interview.

When *family members or close friends* of the client are available in the health care setting, it may be advantageous to *invite them with the client's permission, to participate in the appraisal interview*. Such persons can add an important dimension to the data base, since people close to the drinker often more accurately perceive the full extent of the client's drinking than the drinker does. On the other hand, some family members or friends tend to overcommunicate during the interview, extensively answering questions for the client. In such instances the client has limited opportunity to reveal how he perceives his condition. Obviously it requires additional interviewing skills to obtain a desirable level of participation from both the client and another person, and such an approach need not be attempted until the nurse is skillful in interviewing the client alone. Separately interviewing a person of significance to the client is also an option to consider, but the client needs to be informed and in agreement prior to the nurse's undertaking such an inter-view.

In approaching the client to gain permission to conduct the interview, the *nurse introduces herself and clearly states her professional status*. Once the nurse has made certain that she is *correctly pronouncing the person's name*, she can proceed to *convey the purpose of the interview* and the *amount of time needed to complete it*. The client has a right to know that *he may refuse to answer any question* posed during the interview and that *sharing personal data around certain topics may create some emotional discomfort*. When these aspects have been discussed, *permission to proceed with the interview* may be sought, making certain that the *time selected* to accomplish the inter-view *is convenient to both the client and to the nurse*.

A hypothetical example of how such introductory comments might pro-ceed follows:

Hello, I'm Jane Peterson.

I'm a nursing student from the University presently working on this unit.

Your name is John Smith. Is that correct?

With your permission I would like to spend the next hour with you asking you about your health status in general and particularly how alcohol fits into your life.

This information is essential to plan with you the care you will receive here.

I have a number of questions to ask but want you to know that if you prefer not to answer any of the questions, you can say so and I'll move on to different ques-tions.

It is also possible that talking about some of the matters affecting your health will cause you to feel a little discomfort.

Do you have any questions about the interview?

If not, are you willing to go ahead now with the interview?

While talking with the client, the nurse needs to *pay particular attention to his nonverbal response, level of interest, and any indication of undue anxiety*. It is well to be openly responsive to the person who reacts with annoyance or obvious disinterest to the nurse's request by simply acknowledging the behavior. The nurse might indicate, "you seem somewhat disinterested in talking with me. Am I correct in that observation?" Allowing the person to verbalize any discontent at this point and to clarify the reasons for such feelings will help determine if the interview should proceed or be delayed until a later time. It is essential that both the client and nurse be relatively at ease with one another and in agreement about the purpose and ultimate value of the interview before the questioning begins.

Client interview

There are various styles of interviewing and different methods useful in acquiring appraisal data, all of which can help ensure the success of the exchange between the nurse and client. Although a combination of approaches is actually used with the same client in the same interview, it is useful to separate the approaches when discussing them for purposes of clarity. Styles of interviewing have been identified as empathic, confrontive, clarifying, and advice giving.[2]

Empathy. *Empathic interviewing* conveys acceptance, understanding, and warmth and the sense that one is not totally alone in his trouble.[2] It can bring immediate comfort to the acutely ill alcoholic person who may be immersed in loss of self-worth and in isolation from others. The nurse, in conveying empathy, may respond to the alcoholic person who is sorrowful about deeds enacted while intoxicated by saying, "I can sense the deep remorse you are now experiencing about your car accident when you were drunk last night." Inherent in the nurse's statement is an ability to step inside the person's shoes for a time and genuinely experience pain with him. Although empathic responses are helpful in breaking through feelings that are troublesome, they should not be used to such an extent that the client defers active work on real problems in preference to receiving more understanding.

Confrontation. In contrast to empathic responses is the use of *confrontation*. Confrontation, as defined here, is the act of coming face to face with elements in the interview that interfere with mutual collaboration between the nurse and client. Sometimes in attempting to acquire appraisal data from the alcoholic person, the nurse may experience his lack of motivation for involvement in the process. The nurse may strongly sense that she is "wasting her time" as well as the client's as she repeatedly unsuccessfully attempts to elicit significant data. Or the nurse may feel she is "doing all the work" and that the client is receiving gratification in watching her ineffectually struggle to make a success of the interview. When such a breakdown in communication occurs, the nurse, in an effort to rectify the situation (never as retaliation for the discomfort she is experiencing), can choose to confront the issue head on. Confrontation may range from a puzzled look to a direct statement pointing out to the person the discrepancies the nurse is experiencing. An example of the latter is: "Though you agreed to participate in this interview, I sense that you seem disinterested in answering the questions because your responses are brief and unrevealing. I wonder if you notice this about yourself?" The nurse, in sharing her observation, is attempting to cut through the barriers the client has set up that interfere with the possibility of change. Confrontation in some instances works like holding a mirror in front of the client, enabling him to "see" how his behavior actually looks to another person. On the other hand, confrontation can be seen as a criticism or a rejection, in which case the person may become defensive and more isolated.[2] In spite of this risk it may be essential to use confrontation when the client is undermining his participation in a potentially helpful program of care.

Clarification. When acquiring appraisal data, it is often necessary to *clarify* what the client is saying. The clarifying style involves pinning down specifics about the client's perception of his situation and sorting out one problem from another. It involves the use of a series of questions that, unless phrased tactfully and with interest, can seem impertinent and intrusive to the client.[2]

Alcoholic persons often experience difficulties in focusing their thoughts because of the confusion associated with multiple episodes of intoxication as well as the anxiety accompanying the overwhelming problems resulting from excessive drinking. As a consequence, they may provide vague or unclear responses to questions. If such responses are accepted as given by the nurse, they are useless for accurate and thorough appraisal. An example is the person who answers the question, "How much coffee do you drink during a day?" with "too much" or "a little now and then." The nurse needs to clarify obscure answers by further questions such as, "When do you have your first cup of coffee during the day?" and, "How many cups do you drink at that time?" and then to continue asking pertinent questions until clarity has been achieved. Being persistent and formulating direct, relevant questions that require specific answers are necessary, especially with the alcoholic person who may need to deny problems. As a rule, what, where, when, and who questions are more productive than why questions, since the latter tend to set the person up to provide intellectual responses or alibis.

Allowing the client the time to answer a question fully before posing another helps achieve clarity too. There are times, however, when a client provides prolonged answers or digresses. The nurse needs to interrupt and either rephrase the original question or if it has been answered satisfactorily, go on to a new question. Be sure to ask only one question at a time as multiple questions only confuse the toxic client and unnecessarily force the person to make a choice about which question to answer first.

An additional way for the nurse to be clear in conducting the appraisal interview is to inform the client when she is ready to shift to a new set of questions. For example, the nurse can indicate, "Now I am going to ask you some questions about your heart and lungs." Providing a simple transition statement such as this helps the person make the passage to a new content area.

It is the nurse's responsibility to avoid repetition in questions whenever possible. For example, when the client spontaneously offers information about his present occupation early in the interview as questions appear later in the guide about job status, the nurse needs to build on the prior information. She could say, "Earlier you told me you have been a carpenter for the past ten years. How does being in treatment now affect your employment?" This provides a sense of continuity to the interview and conveys that the nurse is listening to all the person is saying rather than simply attempting to fill in answers to questions on a piece of paper. When the nurse, through the use of a variety of techniques, is successful in assisting the client to pin down and clarify answers to pertinent appraisal questions, she has taken a significant step toward setting the problem-solving process in motion.

Giving advice. A final style of interviewing involves *giving advice*. Although the nurse undoubtedly will find minimal need to apply this style during the appraisal process, its use will be considered, since many alcoholic persons consistently look to sources outside themselves for answers to their multiple dilemmas. As a result, it is common for the nurse to become involved in giving advice to alcoholic clients.

Although there are a number of instances when it is necessary to stipulate directives for the client to follow, especially regarding tangible matters such as nutritional intake, it is essential to understand that giving useful advice about a matter such as alcoholism, with its massive psychologic overtones, is difficult to do. *To be effective, advice must be based on solid theory and a sound understanding of the client's experience, and be free of prejudice.* If offered prematurely, before listening attentively to the client's description of his concerns, advice can be seen as an oversimplification or as degrading. If this happens, advice will no doubt be discarded. At other times, giving advice only perpetuates the alcoholic person's dependence for direction from external sources and does little to promote motivation for self-care. Telling the alcoholic patient to stop drinking or to go to Alcoholics Anonymous may appear to the nurse to be the ideal solution, but if such advice was truly effective, most alcoholic people would be cured.

Finding ways to involve the client actively in determining solutions to his concerns is essential. Brainstorming with the person as to all the possible alternatives and their likely consequences sometimes opens up new proposals for action that are acceptable. Occasionally offering some suggestions about how the nurse might go about handling the situation if she were the client can be effective. The ultimate goal of any advice must be to select ideas that will enhance the likelihood of the client's assuming responsibility for managing personal difficulties.

In addition to styles of interviewing, there are several methods that are of help in acquiring appraisal data from alcoholic persons. Included are giving attention to nonverbal content, to myths and misconceptions, and to aspects of the verbal expressive pattern of the patient.

Nonverbal content. It is especially pertinent for the nurse to attend to the *nonverbal content* of the interview, her own as well as the client's. It is common for the inexperienced nurse to *smile or laugh automatically* when the person talks about matters connected with intoxication. Expressing amusement about drunken behavior is a learned response in our society, where the erratic behavior resulting from excessive drinking is the theme of many jokes. A number of nationally known actors and comedians have promoted their careers bragging about alcohol intake or reenacting drunken behavior to the delight of their audiences. At the same time the alcoholic person may have received positive feedback in the past from others, especially bar companions, for jesting about behavior associated with drinking and intoxication. As a result, he may expect a jocular response from the nurse. Contemplate for a moment what is actually amusing about intoxication. In reality, laughter about the behavior of a drunken person is to make a joke of the toxic, sometimes fatal, response of the body to an overdose of alcohol. Expressing amusement may only encourage the client, who is ambivalent about treatment, to be far too easygoing about serious concerns. It is much more appropriate for the nurse to maintain a serious facial expression and perhaps express empathy for the person's plight, verbalizing the embarrassment the intoxicated client might have felt about drunken comportment. When the client is extreme in using laughter to express his predicament, the confrontive approach may be used. The nurse could say, "You laugh when you tell me about being drunk, and yet drunkenness has resulted in serious consequences for you." The intent of the nurse's response is to encourage the person to begin to acknowledge the severity of his situation and to determine actions for improving it.

Another aspect of nonverbal content during appraisal has to do with *titrating hostility*.[6] Talking openly about drinking can be highly threatening to the client, and this discomfort may be expressed nonverbally, and sometimes verbally, in the form of anger. The main consideration for the nurse is to monitor the client's level of anger continually and to take measures to keep it within tolerable limits so that rapport with the client will not be lost. Two suggestions are offered for accomplishing this goal.[6] *Shifting to a set of questions different from the ones inciting angry feelings may help,* especially if the new questions deal with less threatening content such as physical symptoms. Returning to the original set of questions later may be indicated if the person is calm. A second approach involves the *use of confrontation,* in which the nurse verbally shares her impression with the client that he seems disturbed by the line of questioning. Confronting an angry person obviously requires a higher level of interviewing skill than changing to a different set of questions, and the nurse must be willing to deal with the client's response to her confrontation. It needs to be remembered that the ultimate goal of the appraisal process is to engage clients in the treatment process, not to drive them away.

Myths and misconceptions. *Listening for misconceptions and myths* the client may have about his condition is another interview method. Holding inaccurate information about alcohol-related matters is common in this society and includes beliefs such as black coffee or cold air will sober up a drunk person, a "real" man can hold his liquor, being "high" increases sex appeal, and only skid road people are alcoholic. The latter notion, that alcoholism primarily affects the most depraved, is a widely accepted myth which has kept untold people from seeking help early for their alcohol problem. One patient adamantly proclaimed, "I'm *not* an alcoholic. You've never seen me drunk in a gutter or flopping around with no job and no home."

When the nurse hears the client express a misconception, she needs to take note of it and either discuss it briefly at the time or go over it later after the appraisal interview is completed. Weaving teaching approaches into the history-taking process can be effective in that content is dealt with as it occurs. However, if time is limited or if the client is acutely ill, it may be better to wait until it is more timely to engage him in a dialogue about misperceptions. Allowing ill-founded statements to go unattended encourages the client to retain inaccurate beliefs on which rational problem-solving approaches cannot be built.

Verbal expressive pattern. A final method of interviewing involves *being attentive to the verbal expressive pattern* of the client. Frequently when interviewing alcoholic persons it seems evident that they are reluctant to become involved in the problem-solving process, which is noticeable in the way they communicate verbal responses. Two distinct patterns, discounting and grandiosity, may be noted.[3-5]

Discounting is simply when a person describes something that is significant about the self or another person in inconsequential terms. The vocabulary that accompanies discounting are phrases like, "I can't," "I don't know," "maybe," "kind of," "sort of," and "but."[3] These are extremely passive words that tend to minimize the self. Some people rarely answer a question with confidence and either preface or end a comment with "I don't know—you know." It is as though they have not given themselves permission to think but have assigned others to make conclusive statements for them.

When people use discounting phrases frequently and over a long time period, they end up believing they are true. Such persons also remain in a confused state because of their inability to make a commitment to "yes" or "no." A statement that says "yes, I'm going to stop drinking" is definite. On the other hand, "I think maybe I'd like to try to stop drinking" is a weak and noncommital statement—no one, including the one making it, knows for sure what the outcome will be.

The nurse needs to learn to identify and question the person who uses a discounting vocabulary. When a patient says "I don't know" frequently, the nurse can respond, "You sound so uncertain. Describe the part you are sure about." Or if the person frequently ends statements with "you know," the nurse can say, "No, I don't know, *you* tell me." In so doing, the nurse is helping the client learn to be specific and to search for truths about himself.

A second way of expressing oneself is through *grandiosity*. It is similar to discounting except that the person describes matters in enlarged terms. In the vocabulary of grandiosity the person talks in absolutes, using phrases such as "never," "always," "everyone," "none," or "all the time."[3] These phrases are not only absolutes but gross generalizations. The danger in the overuse of grandiose phrases is that the client, believing they are true, behaves accordingly. The person who says, "Nobody likes me" or "I never do anything right" needs to be asked, "Who dislikes you?" or "Name one person," or "What do you do wrong?" Through such questions the nurse is beginning to help the client accurately assess his situation. If current thought processes of discounting and grandiosity are left unaltered, they can be construed by the alcoholic client as an adequate reason to continue drinking. Also, when these kinds of responses are explored, the nurse may uncover pertinent appraisal data that otherwise would be overlooked.

Reordering the data

On completion of the appraisal interview with the client, the nurse needs to determine if additional sources of data are available: Conferring with other health care personnel as well as studying past health records aids in the development of comprehensive, individualized management strategies.

Finding a quiet environment to think about the interview data gives the nurse a chance to consider her overall impression of the client, his mood, attitude, ability to relate, intellectual and social skills, general level of health, orientation, and ability to provide reliable information. Studying the data in the context of these impressions, the nurse determines the client's activities and demands of daily life and his internal and external resources for meeting daily living requirements. In the process the nurse discovers where imbalances exist in and among these four components. A nursing diagnosis is made for each imbalance, and nursing management strategies are prescribed to correct the imbalances. Sharing and modifying the management strategies with the client to bring them into close accordance with his life-style and goals is essential before implementation takes place. Appraisal is a circular and ongoing process, changing with the client's condition; therefore management strategies need to be monitored carefully and modified when indicated to assure that they remain cogent.

REFERENCES

1. Goldwater, E.: Practical ways to help your alcohol abusers, Medical Times **103:**31, June, 1975.
2. Lurie, H. J.: Clinical psychiatry, Nutley, N.J., 1976, Roche Laboratories.
3. Misel, L.: Personal communication, 1979.
4. Schiff, J. L.: All my children, New York, 1970, Pyramid Publications, Inc.
5. Schiff, J. L.: Cathexis reader, New York, 1975, Harper & Row, Publishers.
6. Weinberg, J.: Interview techniques for diagnosing alcoholism, American Family Physician **9:**107, March, 1974.

CHAPTER 8

Appraisal by physical examination

Many persons entering the health care system obtain a physical examination either because of a specific health problem or concern or as a requirement for employment. The purposes of the physical examination are health maintenance, including education, counseling, and anticipatory guidance designed to identify and, where possible, eliminate high-risk factors to prevent disease. Additionally, physical examinations are used to screen for a specific type of disease, identify latent disease, and evaluate previously rendered care and treatment.[4] The physical examination is only one component of health appraisal, other components being appraisal by interview to obtain a history and clinical procedures such as laboratory tests and x-ray examinations. This chapter describes the role of nursing in and approaches to physical examination. Situational judgments and techniques of examination are also described. A physical examination process focused on alcohol-associated health problems is outlined.

The conduction of physical examinations by nurses is a recent phenomenon. The examination techniques, which are fairly standard, were first taught to nurses by physicians. As a result, many nurses have learned to elicit and utilize appraisal data much as physicians do. As more and more nurses become prepared to perform physical examinations, the teaching process is being accomplished for nurses by nurses. The use made of information as well as the reason for performing the examination separates a nursing appraisal by physical examination from one done by a physician.

Nurses who perform the physical examination need clarity concerning their area of expertise as well as the ability to identify those findings which require referral to a physician. Nurses determine if there is an impairment in the alcoholic person's health status and, if so, what effect it has on his self-care in daily life.[5] In these instances nurses may independently diagnose and manage identified client problems. There are times when a nurse will function in lieu of a physician and thus be performing a physical examination to diagnose disease. When positive findings are detected, the client is referred to the physician for further appraisal and treatment. Whenever possible, clients are involved in the appraisal process and findings are shared with them in an understandable manner. In many instances this may include educating them to physiologic processes so that they can fully understand the meaning and level of their dysfunction.[4]

APPROACH

Although approaches vary, most commonly the physical examination follows the interview designed to obtain a history. Information from the client about particular symptoms and general concerns guides the nurse during the physical examination. A client complaining of abdominal distress, for example, would warrant a more thorough abdominal examination than a client with no such complaint. *Most of the information concerning the client's health status is obtained by interview*. The subsequent physical examination serves to further define and clarify the severity of presenting problems.

The interview sets the tone for the examination. The manner in which the examination is conducted can enhance or destroy rapport developed during the interview. Throughout the interview and physical examination the nurse's demeanor should demonstrate self-confidence, patience, courtesy, consideration, and gentleness.[1] Some clients may be anxious about being physically examined. Reasons may include modesty or fear of the possible findings. The nurse's demeanor can help to allay some of the anxiety, make the client more comfortable, and thereby increase the accuracy of the findings. In addition to demeanor and rapport, evidence of systematic organization on the part of the nurse increases the client's confidence in her ability. A disorganized nurse who does not have all the necessary equipment available, who repeatedly asks the client to change positions, or who is continually moving from one side of the bed to the other may lose the client's confidence.[4] It is also important that the nurse describe what is being done during the examination. The nurse must reassure the client that she will attempt to make him as comfortable as possible throughout the examination. He should be encouraged to communicate any discomfort he might experience.

There are two main approaches to physical examination. One can obtain an entire history first and then proceed with the physical examination, or a brief initial history can be elicited, for example, demographic variables and major symptoms, obtaining more detailed information as the examination progresses. The former approach has distinct advantages in that it allows a substantial period of time for the client to become comfortable with the nurse, the nurse can take notes as relevant material is presented, and the client can remain dressed and in a comfortable position as the interview proceeds. One advantage to integrating the interview and physical examination is that each system can be focused on as a unit and in depth. The choice of styles partly depends on which one the nurse likes best and the condition of the client. Those who are ill or debilitated lose energy quickly. Consequently, it is especially important for them that the nurse develop a system of examination that requires the least number of position changes.

In ambulatory settings the client walks into the room where the examination is to take place and is seated during the interview. The nurse sits directly across from the patient to have an unobstructed view for appraisal purposes. (When the client is recumbent, the nurse should be positioned at his right side.) After the interview the client undresses and is examined. The nurse's hands and equipment should be warmed before touching him. Such thoughtfulness will enable him to stay as physically relaxed as possible. When the examination is completed, the client dresses and discusses diagnoses and management strategies with the nurse.

Equipment for a physical examination includes the following[1]:

1. Otoscope and ophthalmoscope
2. Pocket flashlight
3. Tongue depressors
4. Ruler and flexible tape measure, in centimeters
5. Thermometer
6. Watch with a second hand
7. Sphygmomanometer
8. Stethoscope with a diaphragm and bell
9. Gloves ⎫
10. Lubricant ⎬ for rectal and vaginal examination
11. Pelvic examination supplies
12. Guaiac paper
13. Reflex hammer
14. Tuning fork, 1024 cycles per second
15. Safety pins
16. Cotton (can be cotton-tipped applicators)
17. Paper and pen or pencil
18. Appropriate drapes
19. Necessary slides for specimens

SITUATIONAL JUDGMENTS IN EXAMINATION

To be useful in appraisal, a physical examination must be adapted to the condition of the client, including whether he is intoxicated, withdrawing, or recovering from alcoholism. A complete examination is not always indicated. As has been mentioned, partial examinations may be sufficient and are probably more often employed for routine appraisal purposes, especially when information gleaned from the history indicates few, if any, physical complaints. Keeping in mind what information is required as well as the condition of the client will help in making decisions about how to proceed.

Intoxication

It may be impossible to do more than a partial examination on an intoxicated person, depending, of course, on the level of intoxication. In cases of extreme intoxication it is crucial to screen for any evidence of trauma and acute or chronic health problems that may be exacerbated by intoxication or neglect. More subtle aspects of health appraisal can be deferred until the client is sober. No matter how extreme or inappropriate the behavior of the intoxicated client, overt negative reactions by the nurse are not helpful. Distaste or annoyance, if present, must not be communicated to the client. Although such feelings may be inevitable, it is best to express them elsewhere, perhaps with a professional colleague, with the goal of determining constructive responses. When the nurse is calm, assertive, self-assured, and nonjudgmental, the examination will more likely proceed in an orderly fashion.

Withdrawal

A person in the throes of alcohol withdrawal may also warrant a partial examination because the client is likely to become easily fatigued. Extreme tremors, diaphoresis, or hallucinations can make the actual examination process difficult if not impossible. On the other hand, the nurse might encounter a client who has been sedated to alleviate withdrawal symptoms. With such a client, reactions in general and those to pain in particular may be masked, making appraisal difficult. In these situations a survey for acute or potentially acute problems is essential and often all that can be accomplished. A helpful tool is the Guide for Quick Appraisal of Impending Withdrawal and Emergency Conditions in Intoxicated and/or Alcoholic Persons (p. 106).

Examination of an intoxicated or withdrawing client can be difficult, and is of necessity a shortened process. There is no excuse, however, for an examination that is so superficial as to put the client's life in jeopardy because of neglect. The status of intoxicated and withdrawing persons changes rapidly, requiring that initial appraisals be followed up and reevaluated. One particular client, for example, hemorrhaged severely and died because health personnel assumed he was sleeping off his intoxication after their cursory examination indicated no obvious problem. In fact, he was bleeding rectally, which was missed because no one checked his pulse, blood pressure, or level of consciousness or quickly inspected his entire body throughout the night. This example illustrates the necessity of continually reevaluating intoxicated and withdrawing clients for the possible emergence of acute physiologic crises.

Recovery

A complete examination can be performed on a recovering alcoholic person and is recommended at the beginning of the rehabilitation period. Information gained from such an examination can be used to educate the client about any alcohol-associated physiologic changes as well as aspects important to recovery. It provides baseline data that can be useful in planning for care of the recovering alcoholic person. This examination might also uncover some subtle physical problem that could be dealt with during the treatment process to enhance the client's chances for total rehabilitation, for example, vision or hearing difficulties. Furthermore, data can be used in evaluating improvement in health status subsequent to alteration in patterns of excessive drinking. Lastly, and of special significance to nursing, data can also be used in determining if the client has sufficient internal resources to manage daily activities and what assistance in the form of external resources may be required. These latter questions, of course, must also be posed for clients in acute states of intoxication and withdrawal.

TECHNIQUES OF EXAMINATION

The skills that contribute to the art of physical examination are inspection, palpation, percussion, and auscultation. "*Inspection* is the act of concentrating attention to the thorough and unhurried visualization of the client."[4] It also includes listening to any sounds and paying attention to any odors emanating from the client.

Palpation is the act of touching and pressing, which augment data gathered by inspection. Touch can further delineate information as to masses, organs, joints, temperature, motion, fluid, texture, and moisture. The finger pads are most sensitive; the fingertips should not be used. Fingernails should be trimmed so as not to cause the client unnecessary discomfort.

Percussion is the act of striking one object against another to produce a shock wave that causes vibration. The examiner places the nondominant hand, with fingers slightly spread apart, against the client's body surface and strikes the distal interphalangeal joint with the middle finger of the dominant hand. The blow must be delivered crisply and sharply. Wrist action determines the speed and force of the blow. The motion should be quick and the striking finger rapidly removed from the joint so as not to dampen sound. Fist percussion is striking the dorsum of one hand with the other hand in a fisted position. The purpose of this kind of percussion is to elicit sensation by the vibration of the tissue.[4] The most common applications are to stimulate pain or tenderness to appraise for hepatitis, cholecystitis, or kidney disease.

Auscultation is the process of listening for the sounds produced by the human body. Important sounds are those of (1) the thoracic or abdominal viscera and (2) the movement of blood in the cardiovascular system.[4] A stethoscope with both a diaphragm and bell is essential for appraising the full range of sounds produced under various physiologic conditions.

GENERAL SURVEY

From the time the nurse first introduces herself to and shakes hands with the client, and throughout the interview, she is appraising him and noticing his general appearance, unique characteristics, apparent state of health, and any functional disabilities. The scope of the subsequent interview and physical examination are set at this time. As has been stated, if the client is acutely ill, as for example in an advanced state of alcohol withdrawal, the examination process will be shortened.

The process that will be described is complete and one that would be undertaken in nonacute situations. Height and weight are measured initially. During this time the nurse can appraise the alcoholic person as a whole with regard to body build and bodily proportions, posture, skin color, motor activity, gait, dress, grooming, personal hygiene, facial expression, speech, state of awareness, manner, mood, and relationship to surroundings. After appraising the person as a whole, the focus changes to separate body systems.

BODY SYSTEMS' APPROACH TO EXAMINATION

One particular examination sequence, cephalocaudal, will be described. It is not the only possible sequence. Order to examination is essential, but the particular order is a matter of individual preference. What is important is

Table 5. Alcohol-associated skin alterations with some etiologic factors

Alteration	Etiology
Pigmentation (dirty gray to yellow)	Liver disease
Lesions	Trauma
Abrasions	Trauma
Scars	Trauma; suicide attempt
Spider angiomas	Liver disease
Ecchymosis, hematomas	Platelet deficiency; trauma; liver disease with low prothrombin levels
Decreased axillary and pubic hair	Pituitary dysfunction; liver disease
Fingernail clubbing	Alcoholic cardiomyopathy
Tattoos	Often incurred during intoxication
Diphtheria	Secondary to poor nutritional status, poor personal hygiene, and unsanitary living conditions
Infection	Poor personal hygiene
Ulcerations	Poor nutritional status
	Leukopenia
	Altered circulatory status
Pediculosis	Unsanitary living conditions
	Poor personal hygiene
Scratch marks	Generalized pruritus secondary to liver disease
Palmar erythema	Liver disease

that the examination be comprehensive and elicit all data needed in a particular situation. Each examiner should have a fairly standard routine that allows for smooth and efficient client appraisal without forgetting important steps. Although it is useful to appraise according to the body systems format initially, the experienced examiner organizes and integrates the components of the physical examination by anatomic area.

In this discussion, body system changes related to alcoholism will be emphasized throughout the chapter. Standard physical examination texts can be consulted for more detailed information about specific examination techniques and various pathologic findings. Two particularly useful texts are *Health Assessment*[4] and *A Guide to Physical Examination*.[1]

Skin

Much of the appraisal of the skin takes place by means of inspection when the vital signs are taken. The examiner needs to make certain, through mental review, that all aspects of the appraisal of the skin have been observed. General aspects of the skin that need to be appraised are texture, color, moisture, mobility, turgor, and edema. The inspection of the skin may be the first indication of alcohol-associated physiologic changes, which can be further delineated as the physical examination progresses. A number of skin changes are associated with alcoholism, including tattoos, color changes, and vascular and traumatic lesions. The changes and etiologic factors are presented in Table 5.

Head and face

In examining the head, the size and shape of the skull and condition of the scalp and hair are appraised by means of inspection and palpation. It is important to part the hair at several spots to visualize the scalp more thoroughly. To augment inspection, it is important to question the patient carefully about previous head trauma and to ask about and look for signs of tenderness that occur during palpation. During inspection of the head it is a good time to observe for body lice, which are a major problem for alcoholic persons who live on skid road.

In appraisal of the face the examiner observes the facial expression, the color and condition of the facial skin, and the shape and symmetry of the facial structures, including the eyebrows, eyes, nose, mouth, and ears. Cranial nerves innervating the face may be evaluated at this time but will be discussed with the neurologic system.

Since alcoholic persons are often involved in fights, it is important to palpate the orbital ridges, the bony areas around the eyes, for evidence of fracture that can cause compression of the trigeminal nerve. Palpation of the skull is required to note signs of trauma that may suggest intracranial injury such as subdural hematoma. *Alcoholic persons may have lesions, scars, or masses on the head consequent to accident or trauma that may also cause pain.* Nurses might also diagnose headache or tissue injury secondary to fracture. Loss of consciousness, evidence of fracture, and suspicion of increased intracranial pressure require referral to a physician for further appraisal and diagnosis.

Eyes

Inspection is the examination technique used for appraisal of the eye. *The sclera are inspected for icterus (jaundice), a sign of liver disease as well as other diseases, such as gallstones.* Scleral icterus may be evident before skin jaundice becomes apparent, especially for racial and ethnic groups in whom it may be difficult to appraise for jaundice of the skin. *Conjunctival injection indicates eye irritation, infection, trauma, or recent use of vasodilators, including alcohol and marijuana. The glands of the lids may be sites of infection. Extraocular movements are tested to further evaluate nerve function, which may be impaired due to trauma, alcohol toxicity, tumor, or severe vitamin B depletion, as in the Wernicke-Korsakoff syndrome.*

Pupils are inspected for equality, shape (roundness), and reactivity to light and accommodation. Testing for reactivity to light involves shining the beam of a penlight, which is brought in from the side into one eye at a time. Care must be taken not to shine the light into both eyes simultaneously. A hand placed vertically over the nose between the eyes can help in this regard. The eye toward which the light is beamed is observed for a *direct* response of constriction. At the same time the other eye is observed for a *consensual* constrictive response. Both responses should be present in each eye, but the speed at which they respond may vary. Diminished room lighting facilitates elicitation of this response. *Unequal, sluggish, or nonreactive pupils can be an indication of nerve damage secondary to head trauma.* Clients with nonresponsive or extremely sluggish reactions should be reevaluated hourly and referred to a physician if these conditions persist.

Visual acuity is tested by using a Snellen chart. An ophthalmoscopic examination includes observation of the lens, vitreous body, and retina. This technique requires much practice to perfect and to understand what is being seen on inspection. It is helpful to darken the room to allow for fuller dilation of the pupil. In addition, if the nurse initially closes one eye, visualization is aided. The condition of the vessels and the eye grounds in general yields valuable data concerning physiologic impairment due to, for example, trauma, hypertension, and diabetes. Diligent practice of ophthalmoscopic techniques pays off by allowing the nurse to appraise client welfare in a more complete manner. A summary of alcohol-associated eye alterations and etiologic factors is presented in Table 6.

Table 6. Alcohol-associated eye alterations with some etiologic factors

Alteration	Etiology
Scleral icterus	Liver disease
Conjunctival injection	Vasodilation secondary to alcohol ingestion
Infections	Poor personal hygiene, leukopenia, poor nutritional status, altered circulatory status
Nystagmus	Head trauma, alcohol toxicity, tumor, severe vitamin B depletion
Unequal and/or sluggish pupils	Head trauma, alcohol toxicity
Diminished visual acuity	Preoccupation with alcohol results in neglect both in obtaining eye examinations and in replacing glasses or contact lenses that may be lost or broken

Ears

The ear is inspected for signs of infection and trauma. Inspection of the pinna (auricle) and meatus is made to identify abnormalities in structure as well as inflammation, discharge, and exudate. The otoscope is used to view the ear canal and tympanic membrane. *The canal is inspected for the presence of cerumen, foreign objects, lesions, redness, blood, and exudate. The latter three may indicate infection or trauma.* The tympanic membrane gives significant information about the condition of the middle ear. The examiner needs to be familiar with the landmarks. Bulging or retraction of the tympanic membrane and blood or cerebrospinal fluid in the canal are abnormal, and the client should be referred to a physician for further evaluation.

Auditory acuity may be simply tested by moving a ticking watch from a distance toward the client's ear, asking him to say when he hears it and then repeating the procedure on the other side. This test necessitates a quiet environment. If the distance from each ear is unequal or the client does not hear the watch until it is nearly touching his ear, further evaluation is required. The Rinne and Weber tests further assess auditory acuity.[1,4] These are tuning fork tests, which are useful in determining whether the client has a conductive or perceptive hearing loss. *Alcoholic persons may have hearing loss secondary to trauma or infection or their having ignored* difficulties with their ears when drinking.

Nose

The contour of the nose is inspected for any deviations in shape, size, or color. An otoscope with a short, broad nasal speculum is required for internal examination of the nose. Increased redness of the mucosa indicates infection; pale, boggy turbinates are typical of allergy. *Many alcoholic persons have sustained fractures of the nose and thus will have a deviated and, less frequently, a perforated septum.*

Mouth and pharynx

Examination of the structures in the mouth and pharynx includes an appraisal of the lips, teeth, gums, tongue, mucosa, uvula, and tonsils. As with examination of the head and face, the cranial nerves that innervate the mouth and pharynx may be appraised at this time but will be discussed in the neurologic section. The examination of the mouth and pharynx is conducted from the anterior to the posterior areas of the mouth and begins with the external components of the mouth and jaw.[4]

The lips are inspected for symmetry, color, edema, or surface abnormalities such as leukoplakia, tumor, or cheilosis (fissures at the corner of the mouth due to riboflavin [vitamin B_6] deficiency), and the buccal mucosa for color, nodules, ulcers, and pigmentation.[4] The teeth are inspected for caries, missing teeth, teeth restoration, malocclusion, shape, and tenderness. Typically, the teeth of chronic alcoholic persons are in poor repair largely because of poor oral hygiene and the low priority that alcoholic persons give to dental visits. When they are drinking, the condition of their teeth is of minor concern. Lack of mouth care also contributes to gum disease. The gums are inspected for retraction, inflammation, consistency, and bleeding. *Painful teeth or gums can severely interfere with the daily living activity of eating, which if inadequate, results in deficiencies of internal resources such as energy, stamina, and the ability to ward off disease.*

The examination of the tongue begins with the inspection of the dorsum for any swelling, ulceration, coating, or variation in size, color, or position.[4] The ventral surface is inspected for varicosities or swelling. A purple, cyanosed discoloration of the tongue and its vertical furrow indicates a chronically congested liver. Clinical evidence of vitamin deficiencies often appears on the tongue. A smooth, red tongue, for example, without the normal papillae, is indicative of vitamin B_{12}, B_6, or iron deficiencies.[4] *Alcoholic persons are particularly susceptible to vitamin deficiencies.*

The palate and uvula are inspected with the client's head tilted back. A tongue depressor may be needed to depress the base of the tongue to allow for full visualization. The hard and soft palate, the uvula, tonsils, and posterior pharynx are inspected. Their color and symmetry, evidence of exudate, lesions, edema or ulceration, other signs of inflammation, and tonsillar enlargement are noted.[1] The hard palate is an excellent place to inspect for jaundice in black persons. *Alcoholic persons in general are at risk for the development of oral cancer.* Any evidence of unexplained growth, color change, or ulceration requires referral to a physician for further evaluation. A summary of alcohol-associated alterations of the mouth and pharynx is presented in Table 7.

Table 7. Alcohol-associated alterations of the mouth and pharynx with some etiologic factors

Alteration	Etiology
Cheilosis	Vitamin B_6 deficiency
Caries; missing teeth; retracted, inflamed, bleeding gums	Poor oral hygiene and low priority given to dental visits when drinking
Purple, cyanosed discoloration of tongue	Chronically congested liver
Red, smooth tongue	Vitamin or mineral deficiencies
Jaundice of hard palate	Liver disease
Cancer	? Probable synergistic effect with smoking

Neck

The neck should be inspected for color, texture, scars, masses, symmetry, range of motion, and visible pulsations. The thyroid, trachea, carotid arteries, muscles, jugular veins, and lymph nodes are palpated. Tender nodes suggest inflammation. *Alcoholic persons with cardiomyopathy have increased venal pressure due to congestive heart failure, resulting in distended jugular veins.*

Chest and back

For an examination of the chest and back, the client must be undressed to the waist. The general approach to examination is to compare one side with the other and work from the top down. Examine the posterior thorax while the client is sitting with his arms folded across his chest or at his side and the anterior thorax and lungs while the client is lying on his back or sitting.

Inspect the shape and symmetry of the client's chest, estimating the anteroposterior diameter in relation to the lateral diameter.[1] *As a result of smoking, alcoholic persons may be at risk for emphysematous changes in the lungs, which lead to an increased anteroposterior diameter.* Decreased diaphragmatic excursion is also seen routinely.

Palpation of the chest is used to (1) further appraise abnormalities suggested during the interview or observation, such as lesions, tenderness, masses, muscle spasms, or pulsations; (2) further appraise the respiratory excursion; (3) elicit tactile fremitus (vibrations that occur with speaking); and (4) appraise the skin and subcutaneous structures. *Alcoholic persons may have diminished excursion and tenderness secondary to traumatic rib fractures as well as other lung changes because of smoking-related respiratory alterations. Alcoholic persons are also at risk for an increased incidence of infections in general but especially lung infections including tuberculosis.* Changes in fremitus, percussion notes, and breath sounds indicate various types of abnormalities. For a complete description consult a book on physical assessment.[1,4]

Through auscultation, the nurse obtains information about the functioning of the lungs and the presence of any obstruction in the air passages.[4] Specifically, auscultation is used to appraise (1) air flow through the tracheo-bronchial tree; (2) the presence of mucus, fluid, or other obstruction in the respiratory passages; and (3) the condition of surrounding lungs and pleural space.[1] The stethoscope is used to listen to the chest while the client breathes deeply through the mouth. The nurse must watch that the client does not breathe deeply and rapidly enough to hyperventilate. Auscultation, of course, is done in a systematic manner, and one side of the chest is compared with the other. *Diminished and adventitious breath sounds, for example, are to be expected, especially in older alcoholic persons because of their smoking history and its associated risks as well as an increased risk of infection.*

Breasts

The examiner should perform a breast examination on both male and female clients. The actual examination techniques will not be described here and can be obtained from any book on physical assessment.[1,4] Men are often slighted in this regard. They, too, have breast tissue, although less of it, and abnormalities may be present. *Gynecomastia, an increase in breast tissue that is especially noticeable in men, can occur in chronic alcoholic persons with liver disease.*

Every woman should be asked whether she performs monthly breast self-examination. If the answer is no, she may need to be instructed about the technique. If she answers affirmatively, she must be questioned further to determine if she is examining them at the proper time of the month and if her examination technique is accurate. She should be given an opportunity to ask any questions about the procedure or findings. A brief review of the process is often useful even for the woman who checks her breasts regularly. *Alcoholic women may forget to do the examination because of intoxication and lack of focus on health concerns. In addition, they are more likely than an average population to have irregular menstrual periods because of poor nutrition and other high-risk factors to which they are exposed.* They may need to mark a particular time on the calendar to examine their breasts regularly in addition to checking them after each menstrual period.

After examining the breasts, the nurse should palpate the axillary, infraclavicular, and supraclavicular lymph nodes. The client with any abnormal swelling or tenderness in breasts or nodes should be referred to a physician for further evaluation.

Heart and blood vessels

Integral components of the cardiovascular examination include an appraisal of the heart, the major neck vessels, the peripheral pulses, and blood pressure. The radial pulse is usually appraised at the beginning of the examination. The remainder of the peripheral vessels can be integrated into examination of the associated body part; for example, pedal pulses can be checked during the extremity examination. *Tachycardia may occur in a person withdrawing from alcohol* or as a symptom of anxiety, possibly associated with discomfort when being examined.

The blood pressure is usually appraised at the beginning of the examination also. *The risk of transient hypertension is increased in alcoholic persons because of withdrawal reactions, therefore the blood pressure should be carefully appraised.*[3] Measuring the blood pressure in both arms and with the patient lying, sitting, and standing may be indicated.

For the rest of the examination of the cardiovascular system, the client must lie supine and the room must be quiet. When cardiac appraisal is performed, abnormalities should be assessed in terms of their timing in relation to the cardiac cycle and their location in reference to interspaces and distance from the midsternal, midclavicular, or axillary lines.[1] These lines refer to imaginary lines drawn through the sternum, clavicle, and axilla (Fig. 5).

Inspection and palpation of the heart go together. The focus is to detect right-, left-, or combined right- and left-sided hypertrophy.[4] Any pulsations, thrills, or vibrations are noted. *Left ventricular dilatation of a flabby heart muscle is common in alcoholic persons with advanced cardiomyopathy.*[8] If this condition is present, the apical impulse will feel more forceful and thrusting and last throughout systole. Its location will probably be displaced to the left and downward and occupy two or more interspaces (the normal is only one). Usually the degree of displacement of the impulse correlates with the extent of cardiac enlargement.[4] The impulse may also be diffuse and not located in any particular position.

Important determinants of cardiac performance are venous return and filling volume.[4] A general estimate of these conditions can be made by examining the jugular veins. The best estimate of right atrial pressure, and therefore of right heart function, can be made from the internal jugular veins as well as from the external jugular veins, although the latter are less reliable.[1]

The client is in the supine position for examination of the jugular veins. If the veins are extremely distended, it is best to examine them while the client is sitting. No distention is normally visible with the client sitting. With the client at a 45-degree angle, evidence of jugular venous filling should not extend beyond 1 or 2 cm above the level of the manubrium.[4] Distention is evident when the client is supine, but it should be minimal. Venous filling volume is an important determinant of cardiac performance. Distention that is excessive is an indication that the right side of the heart is functioning poorly.

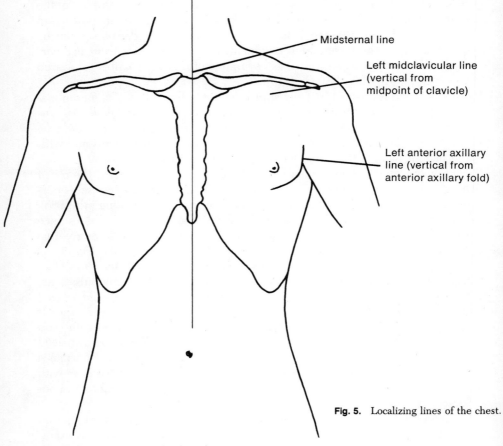

Fig. 5. Localizing lines of the chest.

Anterior

With regard to the heart, symptoms of tachycardia, hypertension, an enlarged heart, and distended jugular veins may be related to the effect of alcohol on the heart muscle. A drinking history is required to establish a definitive diagnosis.

Gastrointestinal system

Essential conditions for a thorough abdominal examination include full exposure of the abdomen, good lighting tangential to the abdomen if possible, and a relaxed client.[1] In addition to techniques described at the beginning of this chapter, relaxation can be achieved by (1) having the client lie

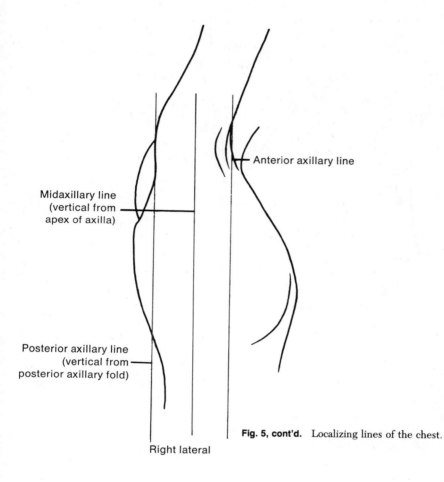

Anterior axillary line

Midaxillary line
(vertical from
apex of axilla)

Posterior axillary line
(vertical from
posterior axillary fold)

Fig. 5, cont'd.   Localizing lines of the chest.

Right lateral

supine with arms at the side, perhaps with the knees flexed or the head on a pillow, (2) having the client empty his bladder, and (3) examining any known areas of tenderness last.

Systematic appraisal is facilitated by dividing the abdomen into quadrants with imaginary perpendicular lines crossing at the abdomen (Fig. 6). As the examination proceeds, it is useful to consider the anatomic structures that exist behind the abdominal wall so as to make some initial judgments about abnormalities.

Inspection is focused on the shape, symmetry and movement of the abdomen and the characteristics of the skin. The nurse should determine if the

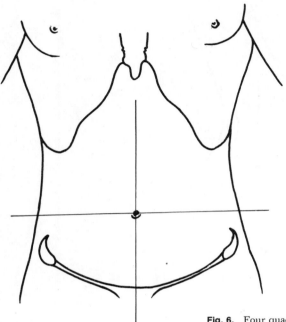

Fig. 6. Four quadrants of the abdomen.

abdomen is flat (horizontal), rounded (protuberant), or scaphoid (concave). *Bulging flanks can be an indication of abdominal fluid retention, which in alcoholic persons can indicate alcoholic cardiomyopathy or cirrhosis.* Tense or glistening skin is another indication of ascites.

Because of its large skin expanse, the abdomen is a particularly good area for inspection of the skin.[4] Observation for pigmentation. lesions, striae, scars, dehydration, venous patterns, and nutritional status may yield valuable information regarding the alcoholic person's general state of health. Jaundice is more readily observed, since abdominal skin is less exposed to the sun and therefore less tanned.

Valuable data concerning previous surgery or trauma can be gained from inspection of the abdomen for scars.[4] If the cause of the scar is not already known by history, it should be clarified at this point. Surgical scars should alert the examiner to the possibility of adhesions, which may make palpation uncomfortable and different from that of most people because of alteration of the architecture of the abdomen. In one instance a particular alcoholic man's abdomen looked like a geographic relief map, showing numerous scars from knife wounds and consequent restorative surgery. In addition, the abdominal architecture was generally nodular from adhesions, resulting in some rearrangement of the normal placement of organs.

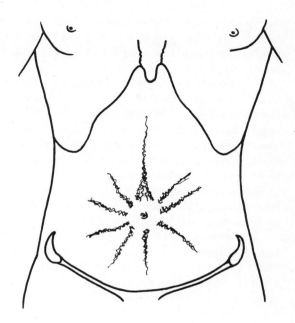

Fig. 7. Caput medusae.

A plexus of dilated veins may be observed about the umbilicus. These indicate obstruction due to cirrhosis and are referred to as caput medusae because their configuration is reminiscent of the head of the mythologic figure Medusa, whose hair was turned to serpents by the goddess Minerva (Fig. 7).

When appraising the abdomen, auscultation follows percussion, since movement or stimulation by pressure on the bowel caused by palpation or percussion is known to alter bowel motility and heighten bowel sounds. Using the diaphragm of the stethoscope, the frequency and character of bowel sounds are noted in all four quadrants. With the bell of the stethoscope the nurse should note the occurrence of any bruits, especially liver bruit, venous hums, or friction rubs. A venous hum is normally heard from the inferior vena cava and its tributaries. In the presence of obstructed portal circulation, as in cirrhosis, an abnormal venous hum may be detected in the periumbilical region.[4]

Percussion of the abdomen is focused on detecting fluid, gaseous distention, and masses as well as appraising the size and position of solid structures within the abdomen, especially the liver and spleen.[4] Appraisal for the presence and extent of ascites can be accomplished by a variety of specialized percussion techniques, among them percussing for "shifting dullness" and the "puddle sign." The reader is referred to standard physical examination texts for elaboration on how to perform these tests.[1, 4] Ongoing monitoring of fluid amounts can be accomplished by obtaining daily weights and abdominal measurements.

Liver size is percussed by beginning near the umbilicus in the midclavicular line (in an area of tympany, not dullness) and progressing upward until the percussion note becomes dull. This spot is marked, and then percussion begins again in the midclavicular line, in an area of lung resonance, and moves downward until dullness is struck again. This place is marked also, and the distance between the two marks is measured in centimeters. The normal liver size in the midclavicular line for an average-sized man is 6 to 12 cm. The liver is smaller in women and short people, greater in tall people. *Since the liver is frequently impaired due to alcoholism, determination of liver size is an important skill in appraising alcoholic persons.*

Palpation is used to explore the abdomen further. It occurs in two stages: light and deep. Before proceeding with palpation; the nurse should check the client's position to be certain that maximum relaxation has been achieved and elicit the client's cooperation in this process. With deep palpation liver and spleen size and condition can be more definitively evaluated. There are various techniques for palpating the liver. Generally, pressure is gradually exerted upward from below the rib cage. Having the client breathe deeply can aid in bringing the liver into a palpable position. *The normal liver edge is smooth, firm, and nontender. Tenderness may indicate hepatitis or other liver problems, whereas the edge of a cirrhotic liver may be hard and nodular. Evaluation of liver size and condition by palpation is an important skill for nurses working in alcoholism.*

Table 8. Alcohol-associated gastrointestinal alterations with some etiologic factors

Alteration	Etiology
Bulging flanks	Ascites caused by cirrhosis and/or alcoholic
Tense, glistening skin	cardiomyopathy
Skin icterus	Cirrhosis
Caput medusae (abdominal collateral veins)	Cirrhosis
Venous hum in periumbilical region	Cirrhosis
Hepatomegaly	Fatty liver or alcoholic hepatitis or early cirrhosis
Splenomegaly	Cirrhosis
Hemorrhoids	Cirrhosis
Gastrointestinal bleeding	Irritation of mucosa, increased pressure in vessels, low platelet count

Also accessible to appraisal by inspection is the terminus of the gastrointestinal tract, the rectosigmoid region. *Hemorrhoids are the most frequent finding in alcoholic persons and can be appraised by inspection.*

It is imperative to evaluate all alcoholic persons for the occurrence of hematemesis; black, tarry stools; or frank rectal bleeding. (Hemorrhoids must be ruled out as a causative factor in the latter condition.) Testing for occult blood by means of the guaiac test is crucial. Pulse, blood pressure, and skin color must also be assessed. A falling blood pressure and an initially rapid pulse, accompanied by paleness and often diaphoresis, may be the first signs of hypovolemic shock secondary to hemorrhage. Early detection of gastrointestinal bleeding is necessary to prevent potentially fatal consequences. Table 8 is a summary of alcohol-associated gastrointestinal alterations.

Musculoskeletal system

Through the history and the previous portions of the physical examination, one can evaluate the client's ability to carry out daily activities that depend on a functioning musculoskeletal system. Inspection includes a comparison of body parts for symmetry and a check for deformities, contour, size, swelling or edema, ecchymosis, or other discoloration.[1, 4] The posture, body alignment, and stance are viewed from both in front of and behind the client. Additionally, the spinal shape is appraised.

Localized joint temperature changes, tenderness, significant changes in shape, range of motion, and muscle tone and consistency are appraised by means of palpation. Muscle strength is appraised by asking the client to move each muscle group against resistance in all directions. *Muscle weakness, pain, or tenderness as well as hyporeflexive deep tendon reflexes may be observed with alcoholic myopathy or peripheral neuropathy.*

Severe hip pain that is unaccompanied by other evidence of arthritis and occurs in middle-aged or older persons, especially men who are heavy drinkers, is suggestive of osteonecrosis.[6] Limitation of leg movement in all directions because of pain will be noted on physical examination. The client may walk with a limp, and pain may be referred to the knee on the same side.[6] X-ray films will usually be negative.

Genitalia

The genitalia are examined according to acceptable techniques that will not be elaborated on here but can be reviewed in any standard physical examination text.[1, 4] Information as to functioning of the reproductive system in general can be obtained by history. *Impotence, for example, occurs more frequently in alcoholic persons. Testicular atrophy is an observable finding in alcoholic men, which in turn results in decreased androgen formation.*

Alcoholic women have an increased incidence of gynecologic problems including amenorrhea. As with other body systems, infections of the reproductive tract are more likely in alcoholic persons.

Neurologic system

Although appraisal of the neurologic system is described separately, the actual examination is incorporated into the appraisal of all the components of the physical examination and interview to obtain a history. For example, mental functions are appraised during the interview process and various cranial nerves during examination of the head and neck. Nursing appraisal of the neurologic system is organized into four general categories: (1) consciousness, (2) mentation, (3) motor function, and (4) sensory function.[5] With these categories, examination of specific parts of the neurologic system can be integrated into the functions they serve. Eating, for example, is regulated by cranial nerves V, IX, X, and XII and can be evaluated by watching the client chew and swallow food. By structuring the nursing examination according to client function, the nurse is more able to interpret appraisal data in terms of effect on the activities and demands of daily living. Specific methods by which to appraise for deficits in functional categories are described here.

Consciousness is appraised as the client engages in conversation with the nurse. Deviations from full consciousness can be appraised by determining the client's arousability and responses to commands and painful stimuli. Abnormalities of consciousness include confusion, stupor, coma, and delirium.[1] A major deficit in consciousness must be referred to a physician for further evaluation. *Alcoholic clients are at risk for alterations in consciousness as a result of, for example, intoxication, traumatic injuries, encephalopathies, and withdrawal.*

Mentation is divided into four functional categories: (1) thinking, (2) feeling (affective), (3) language, and (4) remembering.[5] These components of mentation are appraised predominantly during the interview to obtain a history. The client's orientation to person, place, and time; fund of information; apparent educational level, content of conversation; as well as degree of insight, judgment, and planning are noted. There may be a number of alcohol-related deficiencies in these areas. *An alcoholic person may be disoriented as a result of severe intoxication, withdrawal, head trauma, or organic brain syndrome, for example.* A person's fund of information regarding alcohol can be insufficient for several reasons. Many drinking myths exist, believed by a large percentage of the population, mostly because alcohol is the socially acceptable drug in the United States. Some examples include that alcohol is an aphrodisiac, that one cannot be an alcoholic if one only drinks beer, that drinking can aid in recovery of some infections, particularly colds, and that red wine helps in the formation of red blood cells. During the appraisal process, if the nurse assesses the client's fund of information, she can be in a better position to teach him about alcohol and its effects on the body, focusing on his misinformation.

It is also useful to appraise the degree of insight the person possesses about the effect that alcohol has in his life. The extent of the client's judgment and planning is related. If the client is planning to seek treatment for alcoholism, the nurse can assist with discharge planning by providing treatment options (Chapter 10). On the other hand, if the client does not think his use of alcohol is a problem and certainly does not plan to seek treatment, the nurse would diagnose a different problem and management strategies would be altered accordingly.

Mood, affect, and the client's perception of and reaction to his alcoholism are also elicited during appraisal. *Mood swings are characteristic of alcoholic persons*. Emotional lability may accompany intoxication. Elation is also frequent at this time. Conversely, depression may precede a drinking bout or occur during withdrawal. Perceptual distortions such as hallucinations due to withdrawal may be noted. A strongly intact denial system may interfere with the client's ability to perceive realistically the consequences his alcoholism has for himself and others.

The content and quality of the client's speech, his ability to read, write, copy, name objects, and repeat phrases are also observed. Both recent and remote memory are appraised. Deficits in recent memory can occur, for instance, in persons with Wernicke-Korsakoff syndrome, traumatic injuries, or organic brain syndrome. Also evident in clients with Wernicke-Korsakoff syndrome are mental confusion and an inability to focus attention and fully comprehend reality.

The functional components of *motor function* are (1) seeing, (2) eating, (3) expressing (facially), (4) speaking and (5) moving.[5] While appraising the first four of these, the functioning of all cranial nerves except XI (spinal accessory) can be ascertained. The purposes and techniques to appraise for vision and for cranial nerves II, III, IV, and VI are described in the section on eyes. Horizontal nystagmus on lateral gaze, diplopia, and strabismus are ocular findings in persons with Wernicke-Korsakoff syndrome, for example. Lists of the names of cranial nerves, their specific functions, and tests designed to appraise those functions are available in standard physical examination texts.[1, 4]

Physical motion is mediated by the motor and cerebellar systems. Posture, gait, and position can be appraised when the client walks. *Ataxia is frequently seen in alcoholic persons with cerebellar degeneration*. In affected persons the gait is unsteady and wide-based (the feet are far apart). The feet are lifted high and brought down with a slap. The client watches the ground

Table 9. Alcohol-associated neurologic alterations with some etiologic factors*

General category	Functional category	Alteration	Etiology
Consciousness	Arousing	Loss of consciousness	Intoxication Trauma Metabolic abnormality
Mentation	Thinking	Deficient fund of information about alcohol and alcoholism Lack of insight into alcoholism Judgment, planning for recovery negligible	Intoxication Denial Lack of education
	Feeling (affective)	Mood swings Elation, depression, emotional lability	Intoxication Withdrawal
	Remembering	Deficits in recent memory	Wernicke-Korsakoff syndrome Trauma Organic brain syndrome
		Inability to focus attention	Wernicke-Korsakoff syndrome
Motor function	Seeing (C.N. II, III, IV, VI)	Poor eyesight Pupillary abnormalities Nystagmus	(See Table 6) Intoxication Wernicke-Korsakoff syndrome Intoxication
	Moving (motor and cerebellar systems)	Ataxia, positive Romberg test	Peripheral neuropathy Cerebellar degeneration
		Tremor	Withdrawal; asterixis
		Loss of coordination	Cerebellar degeneration
		Hyperreflexia Hyporeflexia	Withdrawal Peripheral neuropathy
Sensory function	Hearing	Loss	See p. 145
	Feeling (sensory pathways)	Diminished sensation	Peripheral neuropathy—"stocking-glove" type

*Modified from Mitchell, P. H., and Irvin, N. J.: Journal of Neurosurgical Nursing **9**:23, March, 1977.

to guide his steps. He cannot stand steadily with feet together when his eyes are closed (positive Romberg test).[1] Since these findings also occur with peripheral neuropathy, referral to a physician is necessary for differential diagnosis.

Muscle tone, mass, and strength are evaluated during appraisal of the musculoskeletal system. The presence or absence of involuntary movements of the extremities should be noted, for example, tremor during withdrawal or asterixis (liver flap). Coordination can be appraised by having the client walk across the room heel-to-toe and noting any difficulties with balance. Other tests for coordination include having the client run his heel down his shin, watching the client during dressing to see how buttons and zippers are manipulated, and asking him to perform rhythmic alternating movements with his hands, for example, patting his leg as fast as he can or turning his hand over and back as rapidly as he can.

Tendon reflexes can be appraised to add information regarding the risk of complications of motor disability. With the client relaxed and limbs positioned so that the muscle is mildly stretched, the nurse strikes the tendon briskly with a reflex hammer, producing a sudden additional tendon stretch.[1] The client's limbs should be positioned symmetrically and the two sides compared. The reflexes most often appraised are the biceps, triceps, brachioradialis, knee, ankle, and plantar. Reflexes are graded on a 0 to 4+ scale with 0 being no response, 4+ brisk response, and 2+ average or normal. *Hyperreflexia is common during alcohol withdrawal.* However, peripheral neuropathy results in diminished or absent reflexes.

More cranial nerves are appraised while testing the *sensory functions* of smelling (I), blinking (V), and hearing (VII). The ability to detect odors is not a routine part of a screening examination. Blinking is tested by eliciting the corneal reflex. Testing the ability to hear was described in the section on ears. The ability to feel (sensory pathway) is appraised by asking the client when he feels the vibration of a tuning fork applied to the bony prominences of the fingers and toes and then moved medially along the long bones. Responses to temperature, light pin prick, or a cotton-tipped applicator are other ways to evaluate sensory function. *These tests are important when examining an alcoholic client to evaluate the presence and degree of peripheral neuropathies.* Vibratory sense is the first to disappear as neuropathies develop. The extent of sensory loss should be carefully noted so that risks for dysfunction can be adequately determined and follow-up evaluation accurately monitored. The sensory loss tends to be of the "stocking-glove" type. As the sensory symptoms progress, motor signs including loss of strength, weakness, and atrophy of muscles occur and progress slowly over several weeks. Table 9 summarizes alcohol-associated neurologic alterations.

ALCOHOL-ASSOCIATED LABORATORY TEST ABNORMALITIES

The results of a number of laboratory tests are altered by alcohol. The major ones are listed as diagnostic indicators in Table 1 (pp. 16 and 17), under Minor criteria, Laboratory tests. Other tests are used as additional evidence of excessive alcohol ingestion. A summary of alcohol-associated laboratory test abnormalities with pathophysiologic mechanisms is presented in Table 10.

Some of these abnormalities, for example, macrocytosis, are so common in alcoholic persons that if their pathogenesis comes to be understood, they could be used as screening tests for alcoholism. A biochemical test for alcoholism based on the measurement of plasma alpha-amino-N-butyric acid relative to leucine is being investigated.[7] This test, in combination with gamma glutamyl transpeptidase (GGTP) determinations, provided a sensitive means of detection (81% positive) for chronic alcohol consumption with a minimum of false-positive determinations (2%).[7]

USE OF PHYSICAL EXAMINATION DATA BY NURSES

After acquiring appraisal data, the nurse must record these findings for them to be continually useful to others. She must make decisions about what problems must be referred to a physician and what she may manage herself. For the latter the nurse will derive nursing diagnoses and management strategies. Detailed examples of this process are given in Chapter 9. Brief examples common to alcoholic persons are described in this section.

The summation of findings should proceed in a manner similar to the sequence of the examination, cephalocaudal, as well as the techniques used. In the latter instance the most usual order is inspection, palpation, percussion, and auscultation. Sketches can be useful in communicating. For example, the location, sizes, and shapes of scars are best described by drawing the body part on which the landmarks are shown and the dimensions of the scar noted in centimeters. A summary of general observations of the client should precede more detailed information. This summary should be sufficiently specific so that a colleague could pick out the client described in a crowded room. The writing should be systematic, clear, and concise. The nurse reviews the documented findings to diagnose and plan for managing identified problems effectively, as illustrated briefly in the following examples. The diagnosis and management strategies will likely differ greatly, depending on whether the client is in withdrawal or well-established recovery.

On the basis of appraisal of an alcoholic person's skin, a nurse could diagnose, for example, malnutrition, irritation, inadequate personal hygiene, and infections. Any one of these may contribute to imbalances in the client's life, interfering with daily functioning or resources available to meet daily living requirements. If alcoholic persons are malnourished, for example, not only will they experience fatigue and a lack of energy with which to conduct daily affairs but they will also be less able to achieve any additional expectations imposed on them. Malnutrition implies inadequate internal resources in that nutrients necessary for body functioning are lacking. External resources will be needed to allow the client to correct imbalances between activities and demands of daily living and available resources. These may include prepared meals or assistance with budgeting money to purchase food.

Impairment of almost any part of an alcoholic person's cardiovascular system can have serious implications for daily living. In advanced stages of alcoholic cardiomyopathy, for example, the client may be relegated to bed rest to avoid overworking an enlarged, inefficient heart. Some aspects of day-to-day living will change. Internal resources are diminished, and restriction to bed may isolate the affected person from available external resources. Assisting the person to regain balance may include activating external resources by enlisting other professional help; bolstering internal resources by providing adequate rest, nourishment, and psychosocial support; and counseling the person about how to approach and minimize changes in daily living activities and demands.

Abnormalities in the gastrointestinal system range from mild to severe and pose similarly varying problems in carrying out routines of daily life. Simple gastritis, for example, can pose problems related to eating and thereby maintaining adequate nutritional intake. Advanced cirrhosis with portal hypertension, on the other hand, is usually life-threatening and if recovery does take place, the illness diminishes the affected person's internal resources to nearly negligible levels. In either case, external resources are required. Antacids or surgical intervention and permanent adjustments in daily activities and demands will likely be required to achieve a new level of homeostasis. Again, it is nurses who are most able to meet the challenges of assisting persons in reachieving balanced lives after either temporary or long-term disruptions.

Neurologic deficits can result in a number of interferences with daily functioning. Loss of peripheral sensation due to polyneuropathies, as outlined in the example in Chapter 1, necessitates alterations in a person's physical environment so that injury can be avoided. Expectations for daily living are altered, too. The affected person must begin to be more conscious of self-care activities; for example, moving about and foot care require a focus of attention not necessary in the past.

Abnormal laboratory values aid the nurse in determining how able the client is to carry out the activities and demands of daily living based on internal resources. Blood cell abnormalities, for example, result in increased fatigue as well as an inability to ward off infection. The client may be too

Table 10. Alcohol-associated abnormalities: blood and urine with some pathophysiologic mechanisms[2,9,10,11]

	Abnormality	Mechanism
Blood		
Glucose	Decreased	Hypoglycemia from inhibiting gluconeogenesis
Magnesium	Decreased	Lack of dietary intake
Lactic acid	Increased	Increased production and decreased utilization
Uric acid	Increased	Competitive inhibition of renal excretion by lactic acid
Potassium	Decreased	Vomiting, diarrhea, "hepato-renal syndrome"
CPK (creatinine phosphokinase)	Increased	Myopathy due to trauma, ischemia/infarction or hypophosphatemia
PO$_4$ (phosphate)	Decreased	? Renal tubular dysfunction
Serum osmolality	Increased	Reflects blood alcohol levels Every 22.4 increase over 200 mOsm/liter reflects 50 mg/100 ml alcohol
Triglycerides	Increased	?
Cholesterol	Increased	?
Folate	Decreased	Reduced dietary intake and injury to intestinal mucosa
Hemoglobin	Anemia	Folate deficiency, blood loss, liver disease, hemolysis
Red cell morphology	Numerous	Folate deficiency, blood loss, liver disease, hemolysis
White blood cell count	Decreased	Folate deficiency
Differential	Hypersegmented poly-morpho-nuclear leuko-cytes	Folate deficiency
Platelet: count	Decreased	Folate deficiency
Platelet: function	Decreased	Probable interference with aggregation
Mean corpuscular volume especially in 44- to 66- year age group	Increased	?

Table 10. Alcohol-associated abnormalities: blood and urine with some pathophysiologic mechanisms[2,9,10,11]—cont'd

	Abnormality	Mechanism
SGPT (serum glutamic pyruvic transaminase)	Increased	
SGOT (serum glutamic oxaloacetic transaminase)	Increased	
BSP (sulfobromophthalein)	Increased	
Bilirubin	Increased	Direct or indirect
LDH (lactate dehydrogenase)	Increased	liver cell damage
AP (alkaline phosphatase)	Increased	
AMY (amylase)	Increased	
Serum A/G (albumin-to-globulin ratio reversal)		
Vitamin B_{12} concentration	Decreased	
Urine		
Sediment	Abnormal	?
Specific gravity	Decreased	Diuresis; renal tubular damage
Urobilinogen	Increased	Liver disease
Ketones	Increased	Complex, including direct cell damage, starvation, vomiting, and diarrhea
Protein	Increased	?

debilitated to do anything besides devote all his energies to physical recovery from an alcohol-associated disease such as cirrhosis.

In general, the data obtained by physical examination are useful in separating acute (life-threatening) from chronic problems. Acute problems, of course, need to be treated immediately and usually require referral to a physician. Problems of a more long-term nature are often those most amenable to nursing intervention. Changes in activities and demands of daily living and the resources to meet them are necessitated to cope with chronic problems. To this end, the nurse and client mutually establish both short- and long-term goals. These are reviewed regularly and changed as some goals are met, others emerge, and still others become important. If the original data base is sufficiently comprehensive, follow-up care can focus on identified problems and the goals established to deal with these problems.

It is often immediately after the physical examination that effective patient teaching can occur. As findings are shared with the client, his interest in his body and health is usually piqued; thus he is more likely to pay attention to information given him. The nurse can capitalize on this by talking about any alcohol-related physiologic changes that she may have found and how these can be ameliorated. The nurse can also discuss with the client how the emergence of new physical problems can be prevented by changing drinking habits. Altering activities and demands of daily living may aid in achieving this goal. It is also useful to consider what resources can be employed and bolstered to meet current and future activities and demands.

Time spent in this manner is often crucial to establish a nurse-client relationship that may be vital to the client's recovery. The time taken to appraise a client's daily functioning and resources thoroughly indicates a genuine interest in client welfare. Additional time spent teaching the client about what is happening to him bolsters self-esteem and self-confidence, which are essential components to recovery. The client comes to feel that he must indeed be worth something if another person holds him in such positive regard. Such feelings are an important part of the motivation that is required to persist in making the life-style changes necessary to allow full recovery from alcoholism.

REFERENCES

1. Bates, B: A guide to physical examination, Philadelphia, 1979, J. B. Lippincott Co.
2. Drum, D. E., and Jankowski, C.: Diagnostic algorithms for detection of alcoholism in general hospitals. In Seixas, F. A., editor: Currents in alcoholism, Vol. 1, New York, 1977, Grune & Stratton, Inc.
3. Klatsky, A. L., Friedman, G. D., and Siegelaub, A. B.: Alcohol use, myocardial infarction, sudden cardiac death and hypertension, Alcoholism Clinical and Experimental Research 3(1):33, 1979.
4. Malasanos, L., Barkauskas, V., Moss, M., and Stoltenberg-Allen, K.: Health assessment, St. Louis, 1977, The C. V. Mosby Co.
5. Mitchell, P. H., and Irvin, N. J.: Neurological examination: nursing assessment for nursing purposes, Journal of Neurosurgical Nursing 9:23, March, 1977.
6. Saville, P. D.: Alcohol-related skeletal disorders, Annals of the New York Academy of Sciences 252:287, 1975.
7. Shaw, S., Lue, S-L., and Lieber, C. S.: Biochemical tests for the detection of alcoholism: comparison of plasma alpha-amino-n-butyric acid with other available tests, Alcoholism: Clinical and Experimental Research 2:3, Jan., 1978.
8. Smith, J.: Alcohol and disorders of the heart and skeletal muscles. In Estes, N. J., and Heinemann, M. E., editors: Alcoholism, St. Louis, 1977, The C. V. Mosby Co.
9. Stockdell, G., and Allen, N. C.: RBC volume as an index of alcoholism, Lancet 1:1160, 1978.
10. Tilkian, S. M., and Conover, M. H.: Clinical implications of laboratory tests, St. Louis, 1975, The C. V. Mosby Co.
11. Whitfield, C. L., and Williams, K.: The patient with alcoholism and other drug problems, Springfield, Ill., 1976, Whitfield & Williams.

CHAPTER 9

Nursing diagnoses and management strategies

Thus far in the book we have presented a model for nursing diagnosis and management and detailed information regarding nursing appraisal of alcoholic persons. The model is based on the belief that nursing's primary purpose is to assist individuals and families achieve their highest possible health status so that they may effectively meet the demands of their daily lives.

We will now present two clinical examples whereby alcoholic persons are appraised by history and physical examination. *Nursing* diagnoses and management strategies will be derived from the appraisal data. Diagnoses will be stated to highlight the client's functional disabilities that interfere with meeting the activities and demands of daily life.[1] Only those management strategies that constitute nursing's independent practice will be outlined.[2] The clinical examples are designed to clarify the way in which theory presented previously is translated into practice. We hope that these examples will stimulate other nurses to begin to think and communicate in diagnostic terms when involved in the care of alcoholic persons. Nurses need to record their appraisal data, diagnoses, and management strategies for several reasons: to share information with other professionals to enhance client care; to demonstrate more fully their essential position in the provision of care to alcoholic persons; to derive researchable questions; and to provide a permanent data base to allow for careful evaluation of client progress.

The format used to present the examples is one that might appear on a client's record. The headings and subsequent content for the nursing history data follow the interview format outlined in Chapter 6, Detailed Guide for Nursing History of Persons with Alcohol Problems. Physical examination findings are in a cephalocaudal sequence as described in Chapter 8.

Clinical example A

NURSING HISTORY
Demographic data

Ms. L is a 38-year-old American Indian woman born and raised on the Nez Perce Indian Reservation in Idaho. She is a high school graduate. She has lost 40 pounds over a 2-month period and has had melena for 2 weeks prior to admission. She was initially admitted to a small hospital near her home and within 24 hours was transferred to a public health hospital in a large metropolitan area in a nearby state with medical diagnoses of major gastrointestinal bleeding, hepatic encephalopathy, profound anemia, and thrombocytopenia. This appraisal interview and physical examination occurred 2 weeks after admission, following her transfer from the intensive care unit to a rehabilitation unit.

View of current status

When asked what she wanted help with most at present, she replied, "I wish I'd stop feeling dead."

Family history

Ms. L has been a widow for the past five years since her husband committed suicide. She is the mother of three daughters, ages 11, 14, and 16 years who live at home. She describes her relationship with the two older children as "frustrating" and does not feel she is a good mother because of her inability to control her children's lives. They disobey her frequently and also drink heavily, especially on weekends. Ms. L's parents both died within the past three years, her father in a car accident during an episode of heavy drinking and her mother of uterine cancer. She has two younger, married brothers who live near her on the reservation.

The client describes seeing her father drinking heavily the entire time she was growing up. Her mother was a teetotaler. Her brothers drink but have experienced no difficulties with alcohol. She knows of no multidrug use by either her brothers or children. She states that there are no other significant family illnesses with the exception of her mother's cancer.

Psychosocial history

The client lives in her own home and owns one car. She states she does not feel close to anyone—"I'm not that open." She has worked as a waitress in the past but has been unemployed for approximately ten years. Her sole source of income is her husband's Social Security check. She has no religious or other affiliations. Reporting no hobbies or special interests, Ms. L was unable to say how she spent her leisure time except to drink. She expresses extreme alienation from people, stating "I have no one I can really talk to." She appears very depressed, although she reports never having considered suicide. Ms. L is stoic and solemn, denying frustration or anger. When asked how she deals with distressing experiences, she replied, "I drink to forget." She has not had previous treatment or medication for emotional problems. In general, she acknowledges experiencing repeated failure in living up to her and others' expectations and feels like, "I'm no good most of the time."

Drinking history

Ms. L consumed her first drink as a teenager but states that she never drank much at that time because of lack of money. She is unable to recall when drinking first increased, although it has been excessive since her husband's death. Ms. L states that prior to admission she was drinking three fifths or more of whiskey daily. She drinks alone and if friends visit, she soon asks them to leave so she does not have to share her supply with others. She drinks to escape problems but does not like "to make an exhibit of myself when drinking." Her drinking has caused disruptions with her friends and family, especially her children. She says she cannot keep up with the activities of her teenagers and that the two oldest "come home black and blue and I don't know why." She herself has been beaten several times by a nephew with whom she has drunk in the past and has been arrested and incarcerated while drinking, although she declined to elaborate on the circumstances. She received a "driving while intoxicated" (DWI) citation in the past year. Her one previous treatment for alcoholism took place in a 30-day inpatient treatment center in her home state where she was referred by a local physician. She cannot recall the date of the treatment and resumed drinking immediately on discharge. She has never experienced craving.

A typical day spent at home begins by arising about 7:30 AM to make sure her children leave the house by 8:30 AM for school. She has her first drink shortly after awakening and continues to drink heavily and steadily until bedtime, which occurs about 10 PM. She does not eat breakfast but usually has a bowl of hot canned soup with crackers around noon and eats "whatever the kids fix" in the evening. Her main contacts with others include a short visit from a neighbor almost every day "to talk about our kids." She acquires her own liquor by driving to a nearby city.

General health history

Currently she feels physically weak with minimal energy to expend. Prior to the present illness she recalls feeling "as though I was failing" but did not take measures to correct the situation. Her past hospitalizations have been for a cesarean section, hernia repair, and cholecystectomy when she was 27, 29, and 35 years of age, respectively.

Health history related to body systems

Gastrointestinal system: Ms. L does not remember what her eating pattern is when not drinking because she has been drinking steadily for so long. She has never been on a special diet in the past but is now on a 36-gram protein low-calorie diet. She presently complains of mouth discomfort that interferes with eating. When she occasionally experiences nausea, she does nothing because "It goes away eventually." She is frequently constipated and has noticed a considerable darkening of her stools over the past 2 months. She is slightly jaundiced now but had never been told that she had problems with her liver until this hospitalization.

Neurologic system: Ms. L states that it takes about the same amount of alcohol to get the effects she desires as it has for a long time. On cessation of drinking, she has had tremors but no hallucinations, seizures, or delirium tremens. She has never experienced a blackout. Currently she complains of "pins" in hands and feet, with occasional sharp pains, as well as extreme muscle weakness. She states that she has no problem sleeping when at home but was wakeful for 4 days and nights while in the intensive care unit with auditory hallucinations and periods of mental confusion.

Cardiovascular-respiratory system: She denies problems with her heart or lungs and has never smoked.

Musculoskeletal system: She is experiencing muscle weakness and has had some muscle pain in the past.

Integument: She bruises easily and says, "I always have some black and blue marks."

Genitourinary system: She is not currently sexually active. Her menstrual periods are irregular and infrequent. She is a gravida 4, para III, miscarriage 1. She states that she has never had any urinary tract problems.

Drug taking other than alcohol

She denies drug allergies as well as the use of prescribed or street drugs. She takes about six to eight Bufferin a day, "whenever I feel like it", in response to various kinds of physical discomfort, primarily muscle pains and headaches.

Final questions

Ms. L has no plan to quit drinking, stating, "I never said I would stop." Regarding discharge from the hospital, she replies, "I'll handle that when I come to it." However, she seems somewhat eager to be discharged, indicating that she needs to get home to be with her daughters.

Observations about client

Ms. L's short-term memory of events in the intensive care unit is impaired, but her long-term memory, before hospitalization, is fairly intact. She is oriented. She is depressed, alienated, rarely smiles, and appears exhausted and debilitated. She is stoic in character and focuses on the present. The future is of little concern to her at this time.

She seems to be intelligent, answering questions thoughtfully, with a good vocabulary but without elaboration. Her eyes are expressive as to displeasure, anger, and loneliness. She remembers and calls the nurses by their names when addressing them. She is extremely modest and concerned about her appearance.

PHYSICAL EXAMINATION

General impressions: Overweight, semiobtunded American Indian woman, who looks older than 38 years of age. Is presently unable to ambulate because of fatigue and serious illness.

Skin: Dry and warm with multiple bruises and petechiae on arms and legs. Spider angiomas on chest and back. Slightly icteric.

Head: Normocephalic, without tenderness, lacerations, lesions, rashes. Hair dry, thick, and in need of shampoo.

Eyes: Icteric sclera. Bilateral conjunctival injection. PERRLA (pupils equal, round, reactive to light and accommodation). Unable to follow commands to perform visual field test.

Ears: Canals clear. Tympanic membrane intact. Landmarks visible. Hearing intact bilaterally to whispered voice.

Nose: Mucosa pink. No deformities, discharge, or sinus tenderness.

Mouth: Oral candidiasis being treated with nystatin. Encrustations of old blood and oral debris present. Tongue midline. Dentition poor with several teeth missing. Gag reflex absent.

Neck: Supple. Trachea midline. Neck veins not distended. No lymph node swelling under jaw, anteroposterior triangles, or cervical area. Carotid pulsations equal and full. Thyroid not enlarged.

Respiratory system: No skeletal abnormalities. Respirations shallow at 26 to 34 breaths/min and slightly labored. Abdominal breathing predominates. No clubbing. Nail beds pink. Decreased tactile fremitus lower lobes bilaterally. Because of client's obesity and fatigue, unable to percuss for level of movement of diaphragm or lung sounds in general. Wheezing audible without stethoscope. Expiratory wheezes right middle lobe. Diminished breath sounds and ronchi lower lobes bilaterally.

Cardiovascular system: Diffuse point of maximal impulse at fourth to sixth intercostal space next to left sternal border. 1+ peripheral and sacral edema.*

		Pulses		
			Dorsalis	Posterior
	Radial	Femoral	pedis	tibialis
L	4+	4+	3+	3+
R	4+	4+	3+	1+

Rhythm regular at 93/beats/min. Blood pressure, lying: right, 120/63; left, 110/50 mm Hg.

---

*Scale: 1 = weak; 4 = strong.

Breasts: No discharge, retraction, dimpling, or masses.

Abdomen: Multiple abdominal striae. Old scars from cholecystectomy, cesarean section, hernia repair. Bowel sounds hyperactive. No rubs or bruits. Liver enlarged 18 cm at midclavicular line, palpable 4 cm below costal margin. Denies tenderness.

Genitalia: Pelvic examination deferred.

Rectal system: External hemorrhoids, not presently inflamed; stool positive for occult blood.

Musculoskeletal system: Muscle tone decreased in all four extremities. Able to bend arms at elbows but cannot lift from shoulders because of weakness; left side appears weaker. Difficulty bending knees and unable to lift hips without assistance; therefore range of motion not determined.

Neurologic system: Unable to carry out most daily activities independently because of level of debilitation. Hypoactive reflexes. No nystagmus or diplopia. Unable to feel light touch of cotton on forehead or cheeks but able to feel it on chin. Sensation of pinprick on feet and hands diminished bilaterally. Unable to assess gait. Generalized muscle weakness. Gag reflex absent.

USE OF APPRAISAL DATA

In preparation for determining nursing diagnoses and management strategies, the nurse needs to cogitate carefully about Ms. L's *activities* and *demands of daily living*, the *internal* and *external resources* she has available to meet them, and present imbalances in any of these four components. Identified imbalances can be grouped according to the high-risk areas identified in Chapter 1: Physical health, psychosocial and economic well-being, legal entanglements, and factors associated with the diagnosis of alcoholism. The diagnoses and management strategies for Ms. L will be focused on imbalances she is *currently* experiencing. Although we have chosen not to elaborate on imbalances that may continue to be problematic for her in the future, such concerns are certainly germane to nursing practice as essential components of prevention and long-term rehabilitation.

In thinking about Ms. L and her current needs, it is evident that she is in the recuperative phase of a very severe illness caused by her long-term, excessive alcohol consumption. She is, however, still debilitated and is experiencing a number of difficulties meeting the activities of daily living, such as sleeping, eating, eliminating, socializing, communicating, and exercising. The *daily living demands* that she faces are greatly increased, especially concerning the degree of energy she needs to expend for physical repair. Her chronic low self-esteem is exacerbated by a number of factors, including her present inability to fulfill even partially her mothering role and the continued threat to her extreme sense of modesty imposed by hospital routine.

The *internal resources* she possesses to meet these activities and demands partially are her stoic character and her courageous and cooperative involvement in the process of recuperation. Supplemental to these internal strengths are *external resources* available to Ms. L through the health care system, including its personnel and services, as well as income provided by Social Security.

The diagnoses and management strategies that follow would be included as part of Ms. L's permanent hospital record and would serve as guidelines for all nurses and other health care personnel providing care to Ms. L. The management strategies selected are not exhaustive, and the reader is challenged to identify additional strategies that are important to the achievement of nursing's objectives.

Diagnosis	Management strategies
Physical well-being	
Malnutrition secondary to history of nutritional neglect while drinking	Freshen and cleanse mouth prior to eating.
Anorexia consequent to current alcohol-related illnesses	Provide small, frequent feedings (six/day) of high-protein soft foods, including one serving of buttermilk or low-fat yogurt (to improve absorption and aid in reestablishing normal flora).
Peripheral neuropathy secondary to B vitamin deficiency	Provide low-calorie snacks (soft) at bedtime.
	Give multivitamin and thiamine supplements as ordered.
	Grant special requests for food (considering American Indian background).
	Provide assistance with eating as needed because of her weakness and to make certain she does not choke (gag reflex absent).
	Explain reasons for emphasis on current diet (i.e., physical regeneration, obesity).
Inadequate oral hygiene secondary to candidiasis and long-term neglect of teeth and gums	Brush with soft-bristled toothbrush after each feeding.
	Give nystatin as directed.
Sleep disruption related to hospital routine and effects of alcohol on sleep cycle	Provide opportunities for adequate sleep by not disturbing while resting.
	Explain reasons for emphasis on adequate rest (i.e., physical regeneration).
	Discourage use of sedatives by preparing her carefully for sleep, i.e., warm milk, warm blankets, gentle back massage.
	Position comfortably according to her preference.
	Leave bedside lamp on as she often awakens suddenly as a result of frightening dreams.
Constipation with associated gas pains and distention	Gradually increase residue food intake as tolerated.

Diagnosis	Management strategies
	Increase fluid intake to 2000 ml daily; client readily drinks water when offered. (Monitor intake and output.)
	Offer either hot or iced liquids after meals to stimulate defecation reflex.
	Place in sitting position for elimination.
	Provide privacy while using bedpan.
	Provide prescribed laxative.
	Observe for any signs of blood in stool and do guaiac test on all stools.
Diminished energy related to anemia and chronic alcoholism	Range-of-motion exercises three times a day.
	Gradually increase activity; have client dangle legs and sit in chair as tolerated.
Muscle weakness and pain consequent to alcoholism	Observe for nonverbal clues of discomfort and explore with her presence of pain and what might ameliorate it. Give prescribed pain medication when pain is severe or when other measures to alleviate it fail.
	Massage muscles as part of daily bath and bedtime back rub.
Inadequate pulmonary ventilation	Encourage coughing and deep breathing.
	Change position in bed every 2 hours.

Psychosocial well-being

Diagnosis	Management strategies
Diminished self-esteem related to alcoholism, present illness, ethnic group, and gender	Express empathy, warmth, and friendliness by frequent, short visits when awake, offering her unsolicited care and comfort.
	Emphasize her value as an individual by providing choices and involvement in decision making regarding her care.
	Provide an atmosphere of acceptance by listening attentively and talking with her about her concerns and interests, specifically, the welfare of her children.
	Recognize, without confronting, her need for current use of denial about her alcoholism
	Build on strengths and resources that may be useful in recovery from alcoholism, such as her stoicism; for example, bolster her courageous attitude toward recuperation by identifying with her the daily progress she makes.
Depression, moderately severe, related to physical and psychosocial factors, i.e., re-	Foster pride in appearance by assisting with personal hygiene including hair shampoo and combing.

Diagnosis	Management strategies
lationship with children, alcoholism, current illness	Offer hope about possibilities for long-term recovery.
	Listen carefully for suicidal ideation. If expressed, openly discuss it with her and carefully monitor her behavior.
Extreme modesty in regard to exposure of body	Refrain from performing nonessential procedures.
	Provide ample privacy when using bedpan and while bathing.
	Encourage verbalization of concerns about undesired exposure by discreetly acknowledging nonverbal behavior.
Lack of alternatives to occupy time	Provide stationery so that she can write to daughters.
Social isolation	Encourage quiet, diversional activities suited to Ms. L's interests in collaboration with occupational therapist.
	Encourage socialization with roommate by synchronizing their active times and then placing them in close physical proximity to allow eye contact and card playing.
	Provide reading materials, in particular those related to her own cultural background.
	Contact staff at local American Indian Cultural Center to socialize with Ms. L for short time periods as tolerated.

Economic well-being

Diminished financial resources	Have a member of the hospital auxiliary contact Ms. L to arrange provision of needed personal articles.
	Encourage Ms. L to write to her family and ask them to send a small sum of money to cover incidental expenses.

Legal entanglements

Anxiety regarding driving while intoxicated citation	Enable her to describe those factors which intensify her anxiety over this issue. Use sensitivity concerning invasion of privacy when questioning her about personal matters.
	Clarify that little can be done at this time to resolve the problem.
	Problem solve concerning long-term options.

Diagnosis	Management strategies

Factors associated with the diagnosis of alcoholism

Denial with consequent unwillingness to plan for ways to achieve abstinence

Be alert for opportunities to begin teaching Ms. L how her current illness is related to excessive drinking.

Avoid emotional appeals to stop drinking or moralizing about alcohol and alcoholism.

Discuss need for her to achieve total abstinence and reasons for it, e.g., to halt physiologic damage caused by her excessive alcohol consumption.

Keep any discussions about her alcohol problems focused on present short-term goals rather than concentrating on the future in any depth.

Arrange a conference with any family members who might visit to discuss gravity of her alcoholism problem and their potential role in its amelioration.

Provide written information about AA meetings in the hospital setting. Encourage her attendance when more fully recuperated.

Inform her of availability of local American Indian Alcoholism program that provides motivational counseling as well as long-term rehabilitation. Encourage her to meet with staff representative from this program.

Clinical example B

NURSING HISTORY
Demographic data

Mr. C is a 21-year-old white man born in the Northwest and raised in the Southwest. He finished ninth grade, obtained an equivalency high school diploma, and then attended one year of college. After serving one year in the Coast Guard, he was dishonorably discharged for selling marijuana.

View of current status

Mr. C is currently in the second day of a 28-day residential alcohol treatment program, having been transferred directly from a detoxification center where he spent 5 days. He was referred for treatment by the court after conviction for attempted burglary while intoxicated. Prosecution was deferred in lieu of successful completion of treatment for his alcoholism. Mr. C states that he wants help to "not take a drink even when I want to. I want to be able to run my own life. I can't do that with alcohol."

Family history

Mr. C has never been married. He has two older brothers and one younger sister, ages 28, 26, and 19 years, respectively. His parents were divorced when he was 3 years old, and he has not seen his father since. His mother remarried shortly after her divorce, and the family moved to the Southwest. Mr. C reports that he never liked his stepfather, who drank heavily and was often physically abusive to his mother and older brother and on infrequent occasions to him. In response to this abusiveness, he developed a pattern of running away from home several times a year from 12 years of age through adolescence. He would be gone for as long as a week until the police caught him and returned him to his home. His mother only drank about once a year, but when she did would become extremely intoxicated. When Mr. C was asked what he learned about alcohol when growing up, he replied, "It taught me that I would never become an alcoholic, but I did." He describes himself as the only one of his siblings and other relatives who has alcoholism or other drug problems. There are no major illnesses in his family.

Psychosocial history

Immediately prior to admission and for the past several months, Mr. C had been living alone in a "cheap hotel" in a small coastal city. His means of transportation was walking. Before living in the hotel, he lived with a woman friend in a house in the same city. He feels close to his grandmother who is a nondrinker, a male friend with whom he drank, and a woman friend who is not a heavy drinker.

Mr. C has no special job skills, but has done landscaping in the past for short time periods. He is presently unemployed and living on welfare. He has no active group affiliations and spends most of his time drinking. Past interests from which he has derived satisfaction included collecting coins, hiking, camping, and playing basketball and softball. He says that he feels depressed about once a month for 3 to 5 days at a time, experiences considerable anger and frustration, but "I don't show it," and is nervous "just about all the time." He often feels estranged from others and said, "Sometimes I feel that if I really got into bad trouble, I wouldn't have anyone I could talk to."

Mr. C has thought about suicide infrequently and has never actively planned to carry it out. He usually does not show his feelings, but because of a positive counseling experience with a psychiatrist while in the Coast Guard, he recognizes the value of talking about his feelings with another person.

In general, he acknowledges that since his teenage years he has pretty much wasted his life but now feels more hopeful about the future as a result of being in treatment.

Drinking history

Mr. C had his first drink at 12 years of age in seventh grade, at which time he became drunk and thereafter began drinking to drunkenness on weekends until 16 years of age. He started drinking daily at about this time as well as using other drugs," . . . acid, speed, coke, downers, Quaaludes, marijuana. I used everything but heroin. I heard heroin was so good I was afraid to try it." His favorite form of liquor is beer, and prior to admission he was drinking alone in his hotel room most of the day. However, he states he prefers to drink in taverns with a friend who shares the goal of getting drunk. When asked what initiates his drinking, he responded "Just getting up." He says he is most likely to drink "when I fight with a girlfriend" or "when someone says something to me I don't like." Drinking has caused him to lose friends and one job and to disrupt his schooling. "I just wanted to get drunk and stoned all the time so I quit school in the ninth grade." When he is drunk, he becomes aggressive, fights with others, and "I go around town busting out windows and stealing stuff." He sometimes gives away what he steals and at other times sells it for cash for beer. He has had one car crash when drunk and a broken arm in a drunken brawl as well as numerous cuts on arms from breaking windows when drunk. He was imprisoned for 45 days in the Coast Guard for possessing marijuana. He is currently on deferred prosecution for burglary while intoxicated. Mr. C says he constantly craves a drink since being in the treatment center. He has had no previous long-term treatment for alcohol or other drug problems other than detoxification before this admission.

Prior to admission a typical day was spent in the following way: Mr. C got up about 8 AM and smoked cigarettes until around 9 AM while thinking about getting some beer. He would leave his hotel room and go out on the streets and look for someone to drink with. If successful, he would spend the day going from tavern to tavern drinking beer and visiting people around town. "Sometimes we'd throw a frisbee in the park." If unable to find a drinking partner, "I'd get a supply of beer and stay in my room to drink it." He would retire around 2 or 3 AM.

General health history

In describing his current state of health, he says he feels "tired" and "sometimes I feel like I'm going to pass out." He had one major illness at 19 years of age, when on two occasions for 2 days, he passed bright red blood in his urine. This was treated, but he states that he never understood the diagnosis. He has a history of ear infections both as a child and an adult, occurring about three times a year. He describes "popping" sounds associated with them as well as a yellowish discharge. He had bleeding from his ears during one episode last year. He rarely seeks treatment for these problems, preferring to let them go away by themselves.

Health history related to body systems

Gastrointestinal system: His daily eating pattern when drinking consists of "maybe grabbing a berry pie and carton of milk." When not drinking, he eats two full meals a day. When drinking, he sometimes has stomach pain and diarrhea and notices that the color of his stool occasionally is "black or really light."

Neurologic system: He states that he needs more beer now than previously to get drunk. When withdrawing from alcohol, he has experienced irritability, nervousness, tremors, and "feeling very rundown." He has had at least "ten blackouts in the past two years." He states that he sleeps well and feels rested after 6 or 7 hours of sleep.

Cardiovascular-respiratory systems: He notices that his heart "misses a beat" occasionally, and he is aware of rapid heartbeat "when I get excited." He coughs frequently, raising large amounts of mucus, which he relates to his habit of smoking 1½ to 2 packs of cigarettes a day for the past six years.

Musculoskeletal system: He has had one fracture of his right arm when drunk at 19 years of age. He currently complains of intermittent back pain.

Integument: He bruises easily from "messing around when drunk."

Genitourinary system: He had gonorrhea, accompanied by painful urination, at 18 years of age, when in the Coast Guard. At 19 years he had two episodes of passing bright red blood in his urine. He is sexually active and encounters no difficulty with sexual functioning "unless I'm too plastered" and then is unable to achieve an erection. He uses no form of contraception and fails to ask if his sexual partner is protected against unwanted pregnancy. He states, "I feel guilty about that and guess I'd better figure out what to do."

Drug taking other than alcohol

He says that he does not use any over-the-counter drugs and that he spontaneously curtailed his extensive street drug use several years ago. When using speed, his gums bleed "just from barely touching them." He had bruxism (jaw grinding) and numerous infections at sites of injection from "shooting up."

Final questions

When he completes residential alcoholism treatment, he plans to take Antabuse because "I don't want to go on drinking." He says he will attend Alcoholics Anonymous and be involved in counseling at a community alcohol center. He wants to learn a job skill and is making plans presently to be involved in vocational rehabilitation.

He spontaneously stressed the importance of having some family members involved in his treatment because "if I feel they aren't for my getting better, I may go back to drinking."

Observations about client

Mr. C relates in a straightforward manner, maintaining direct eye contact. His comments are frank and reliable, and he willingly elaborates on each question asked. He is hopeful about the future but also expresses skepticism about how successful he will be in achieving recovery from his alcohol problem. He is of average intelligence and is well oriented. He appears physically tired with a low energy level.

PHYSICAL EXAMINATION

General impressions: Mr. C is a thin young man with sandy-brown long hair and a slightly stooped posture. He exhibits good eye contact and has a friendly manner. He is in no acute distress at the present time.

Vital signs: Temperature 98.2°; pulse rate 88 beats/min; respirations 18 breaths/min; blood pressure 104/70 mm Hg; weight 140 pounds; height 5 feet 10 inches.

Skin: Pale pink with blotchy red-white spots on hands and feet suggestive of poor circulation. Cigarette stains on fingers. Warm to touch; no excoriations but numerous bruises and small healed scars on arms and legs. Athlete's foot fungus present on both feet between toes. Normal hair distribution and consistency. Nail beds pink with normal blanching, no clubbing.

Head: Normocephalic. Hair needs washing. Scalp without signs of injury. No masses. No lesions.

Eyes: Vision not tested. Client reports no difficulty with vision. Conjunctival injection, sclera white. PERRLA (pupils equal, round, reactive to light and accommodation). Extraocular movements intact. No ptosis, strabismus, or nystagmus. Ophthalmoscopic: red reflex normal. Optic disc creamy pink, round, with sharp edges.

Ears: No masses or lesions of auricle. Moderate amounts of cerumen in canals. Canals inflamed, especially the right. Tympanic membrane visualized right, but structures deviated; appears slightly retracted. Scars from previous infections visualized. Left tympanic membrane not visualized. No light reflex. No discharge from ears at present. Response to whispered voice indicates acuity not grossly impaired.

Nose: Patent bilaterally. No deviation. Mucosa pink. No sinus tenderness.

Mouth: Lips red, no lesions. Mucosa pink. Gums healthy. Teeth in good repair but yellow. Tongue midline, reddish smooth surface. Posterior pharynx reddened. Tonsils enlarged. Uvula deviated to right. Gag reflex present.

Neck: Full range of motion. Veins not distended. Carotid pulses equal and strong. Trachea midline. Thyroid isthmus barely palpable, lobes not felt. No lymphadenopathy.

Chest and lungs: Chest symmetric, expansion and diaphragmatic excursion equal bilaterally. Poor excursion. Lungs resonant. Breath sounds without wheezes or other abnormal sounds. Anteroposterior diameter not increased.

Heart: Apical impulse barely palpable between the fourth and fifth left intercostal space medial to midclavicular line. Heart sounds normal. No murmurs, gallop, or rubs detected.

Breasts: Symmetric. Not enlarged. No masses, tenderness, or lesions.

Abdomen: Flat. No lesions. No hernia. No pulsations. Peristalsis not visible. Normal bowel sounds. No friction rubs or bruits. No masses or tenderness, liver edge at costal margin, nontender. Size: 10 cm at midclavicular line.

Genitalia: Normal male.

Rectal system: Negative. Brown stool, negative for occult blood.

Musculoskeletal system: No joint deformities. Normal range of motion, including hands, wrists, shoulders, spine, hips, knees, ankles.

Peripheral vascular system: Both right and left radial, femoral, dorsalis pedis, and posterior tibialis pulse 4 + .

Neurologic system:

Mental status: Alert, responsive, cooperative. Memory and orientation intact for present and past. Appropriate behavior and speech.

Cranial nerves: Able to perform activities of daily living without adjustments to any impairment.

Motor system: Gait normal, heel-to-toe walking good. Romberg test negative. Coordination intact bilaterally. No tremors. Hand grip strong.

Sensory system: Screening for vibration and light touch intact.

Reflexes: All brisk at 2 + .

Impressions: Mr. C is in no acute distress at this particular time. His excessively thin stature and smooth, red tongue indicate the need for nutritional repair during treatment. He will be referred to a physician for further evaluation of his ears. He seems motivated and eager to recuperate and to alter his drinking habits.

USE OF APPRAISAL DATA

As with the former client, Ms. L, the nurse at this point thinks carefully about Mr. C's daily living activities and demands and the resources he has to meet them. Imbalances are grouped according to the high-risk areas previously outlined in Chapter 1. Diagnoses and management strategies for Mr. C are derived from those imbalances which he is *currently* experiencing.

Mr. C has no major interferences in his ability to meet the *activities of daily living* while in an alcohol treatment center. The most pressing *demand* he faces is to remain sober, which presents some difficulty because of the craving he is currently experiencing.

In regard to *internal resources*, Mr. C's youth and the fact that he has *not* had major irreversible physical damage, in spite of his intensive history of heavy drinking, smoking, and other drug use, are to his advantage. In addition, Mr. C is eager to learn about and to discuss his problems frankly and openly. His manner is warm and engaging. Because his excessive drinking was associated with adolescence and early adulthood, the developmental tasks of these stages, including the ability to cope on his own, to make his own living, and to develop meaningful interpersonal relationships, have not been adequately achieved. This developmental delay represents a deficit in

Mr. C's internal resources that must be addressed so that he can meet the challenges of adulthood and recovery from alcoholism more fully.

His *external resources* are limited. There are presently two nondrinking people to whom he feels close: his maternal grandmother and one female friend. A male peer, whose friendship he values highly, is a heavy drinker and thus is unavailable as a resource at the present time. Mr. C has no job or permanent living arrangements, and his income is restricted to welfare payments. The treatment center with its professional services is a viable support system for Mr. C. The ability of the agency staff to assist him with current problems and to provide a transition back to the community are additional crucial adjuncts to his potential recovery.

Diagnosis	Management strategies
Physical well-being	
Potential malnutrition as evidenced by smooth, reddened tongue, gaunt appearance, and low energy level related to diminished appetite and inadequate intake while drinking and smoking	Place on balanced diet with protein supplements of milk shakes and cheese midafternoon and at bedtime.
	Grant special requests for food, i.e., enjoys pizza and submarine sandwiches delivered from nearby delicatessen.
	Weigh weekly.
	Give multivitamin daily.
	Teach the principles of good nutrition and explain the current emphasis on high-calorie, high-protein supplements.
	Provide opportunities to increase physical activity to increase muscle tone and stimulate appetite. Prefers jogging before breakfast every morning.
Backache of undetermined origin, possibly related to tension and/or poor body alignment	Provide a firm mattress and bed boards.
	Offer pain-reducing measures including heating pad, warm baths, nonprescription medication such as aspirin.
	Teach muscle-conditioning exercises for alleviating low back pain, good posture and body mechanics, and factors that exacerbate backache such as fatigue.
	Place in progressive relaxation class to teach him how to reduce muscular tension.
	Ask him to pay close attention to and report to the nurse what is effective in relieving back pain.
Cough productive of large	Discourage smoking.

Diagnosis	Management strategies
amounts of whitish, yellowish sputum secondary to smoking	In-depth teaching regarding hazards of smoking. Give him referral information concerning where he can obtain assistance in stopping smoking. Instruct him to monitor and report to nurse any changes in mucus produced from coughing.
History of recurrent ear aches and discharge from ears	Explain symptoms indicative of ear infection, i.e., pain and discharge from ear, stressing importance of seeking immediate health care when ear discomfort develops. Refer to physician or nurse practitioner for evaluation of current ear status.
Athlete's foot	Instruct him to dry well between toes after showering. Apply Desenex twice a day. As precaution against fungal transmission, have him wear his leather shoes around the treatment center; disinfect shower stall after use.
Sensation of passing out of undetermined origin	Encourage him to evaluate antecedent events systematically for clues concerning possible etiology. Instruct to lower his head and get into a recumbent position when an episode occurs. Give hot liquids and complex carbohydrate foods when symptoms appear. Monitor any change in status associated with these procedures. Monitor effect of learning relaxation skills on frequency of these episodes.
Psychosocial well-being	
Nervousness	Approach unhurriedly. Demonstrate calmness. Arrange a structured, orderly environment with established routines. Evaluate effects of relaxation classes. Listen attentively and talk with him about his nervousness.
Inability to express anger directly Depression Resentments about past family conflicts, especially with stepfather	Observe for nonverbal clues that he is experiencing emotional discomfort, i.e., clenching jaw when in uncomfortable situations, sorrowful appearance and sulkiness; verbalize such observations to him in an atmosphere of acceptance.

Diagnosis	Management strategies
	Emphasize importance of recognizing tension within himself.
	Encourage verbal expression of feelings both with individuals as they occur and in therapeutic group interaction.
	Explain to him how to channel his emotional energy into activity such as physical exercise or pounding punching bag.
Insufficient interpersonal relationships	Place him in social skills training group for purposes of learning how to relate to others in absence of alcohol.
	Have him invite grandmother and female friend to attend and participate in regularly scheduled treatment activities for family and close friends.
	Membership on treatment center's softball team.
	Capitalize on his acknowledged interests and refer him to community groups established around such interests, e.g., numismatics, hiking, and camping clubs.
	Encourage closer attention to personal hygiene, e.g., shampooing
Craving for alcohol	Reassure that craving is most intense during early phases of recovery and will gradually decrease in intensity and frequency as sobriety lengthens.
	Suggest alternatives to drinking when experiencing craving, including participation in specific activities like jogging and reading, eating snacks consisting of protein or complex carbohydrates, and seeking support of other people, especially those currently available in treatment program and in AA.
Guilt related to lack of use of contraception when engaging in sexual intercourse	Determine his degree of understanding regarding sexual matters.
	Encourage him to accept and act on his responsibility for preventing unwanted pregnancies in sexual partner.
	Discuss options for contraception (explain that condom also prevents transmission of venereal disease).
	Advise him about availability of Planned Parenthood should he desire further information.

Diagnosis	Management strategies
Economic well-being	
Inadequate job skills	Encourage participation in vocational rehabilitation program and discuss progress made.
Legal entanglements	
Anxiety related to outcome of deferred prosecution for burglary attempt while intoxicated	Offer positive feedback about his choice of participation in treatment to solve his alcohol problem (which results in criminal behavior) on a long-term basis
	Encourage him to talk about his anxiety over this issue.
	Discourage his perseveration about possible negative outcome of this legal matter. Emphasize that positive outcome primarily depends on his successful completion of alcoholism treatment.
Factors associated with diagnosis of alcoholism	
Perplexed and confused about his developing alcoholism and its amelioration	Encourage him to verbalize related anxieties and to ask questions about alcoholism.
	Provide ample opportunity to clarify misconceptions held and supplement his knowledge through discussion and relevant reading materials.
	Refer to physician for possible disulfiram (Antabuse) prescription.
	Provide with listing of local age-appropriate AA meetings and encourage him to attend at least two meetings a week.
	Begin discharge planning, focusing on halfway house placement while he is completing his job training and until he becomes employed.
	Discuss with him the natural consequences of his aggressive acts while drunk, i.e., physical self-injury and legal problems. Underscore resultant necessity of effectively altering his excessive drinking pattern through completion of treatment and continued involvement in AA, job training, and personal growth activities.

Finally, an important part of developing the foregoing management strategies was mutual collaboration with both Ms. L and Mr. C. This process is vital for all clients, and through it the nurse elicits the client's personal ideas concerning options and preferences for care. The mutual selection of management strategies may take several forms, depending on the mental, emotional, and physical capabilities of the client and family. The nurse and client may actively work together on defining management strategies, or in a different situation, the nurse may need to define the strategies and then ask the client if they are agreeable. If collaboration does not occur, conflict about the strategies chosen may interfere with the client's ability to achieve maximum recovery.

As the nurse implements management strategies, evaluation of their effectiveness and accuracy of the diagnoses becomes an ongoing process. The nurse monitors whether anticipated outcomes are achieved. Prognostic indicators useful in nursing are those which assist in determining the extent to which the management strategies enable the client to mobilize and utilize external and internal resources in meeting activities and demands of daily living to the fullest extent possible.

REFERENCES

1. Campbell, C.: Nursing diagnosis and intervention in nursing practice, New York, 1978, John Wiley & Sons, Inc.
2. Mitchell, P. H.: Concepts basic to nursing, New York, 1977, McGraw-Hill Book Co.

CHAPTER 10

Treatment of the alcoholic person

In preceding chapters, discussions have focused on the appraisal and diagnosis of persons with alcoholism and on the recognition of signs and symptoms that are indices of needs for which nursing actions must be planned. Crucial to rehabilitation of the person with alcoholism are the management strategies derived from the appraisal process. Management strategies must take into consideration the individual's needs, be congruent with his life-style, and hold the promise of leading to improved health and an enriched quality of life. The intent of this chapter is to familiarize the reader with issues involved in planning the rehabilitation of alcoholic persons and to present evaluation of major treatment strategies.

The process of detoxification and the nature of the withdrawal syndrome, viewed as acute episodes of alcoholism that generally precede entry into treatment, are discussed and nursing management strategies during these episodes are presented. Major treatment modalities including Alcoholics Anonymous, counseling, behavioral approaches, and deterrent agents are evaluated in terms of their usefulness toward long-term rehabilitation as are major alcoholism services such as community alcohol centers, alcohol inpatient treatment facilities, and alcoholism outpatient clinics. Last, some elements known to influence behavior in general are reviewed as they relate to an understanding of behavior of alcoholic clients.

THE ENGAGEMENT PROCESS

It is a truism to say that a relationship with the alcoholic person must be established to help him toward recovery from alcoholism. It is often extremely difficult for the alcoholic person to present himself for treatment, which is the first step toward the establishment of a therapeutic relationship. No matter how excessive his drinking and regardless of how disastrous its consequences, the alcoholic person can usually point to others who do not consider themselves alcoholic and who are actually in worse straits. Using such persons as a base for defining himself, he reinforces his mistaken conviction that he is not an alcoholic, is not in need of help, and does not need to change his way of drinking. Other reasons are frequently used to explain problematic drinking behavior and rejection of treatment, including stressful job situations, domestic problems, and ill health. All of these are seen by the alcoholic client as causes of problematic drinking rather than as its consequences.

Engaging the alcoholic person in a treatment program as soon as possible is important. As in any chronic condition, the earlier treatment is provided the greater are the chances for recovery and rehabilitation. When progression of alcoholism is interrupted at an early stage, pathophysiologic consequences are usually reversible, the family unit is intact, and the activities of daily living are less disrupted. Under such conditions, therapeutic interventions are more effective. Unfortunately, while still experiencing a more or less integrated way of life, the alcoholic person is less motivated to acknowledge problems resulting from his drinking or to enter into a treatment program that is aimed at changing his drinking behavior. Finding a way to help the alcoholic person acknowledge the problem early and to accept treatment is one of the most challenging tasks facing health professionals and people close to the alcoholic person, all of whom usually have recognized and diagnosed alcoholism long before the affected person can accept it.

As is probably true for most persons facing the need for change, the alcoholic person ultimately acts in response to some form of coercion, whether it involves the threat of a divorce, the loss of a job, repeated encounters with the law, or recognition that physical health is deteriorating. At such times the person may enter an alcoholism treatment program or look for help from nurses, physicians, friends, ministers, or social workers. Even then, the reasons given for seeking help may be other than to receive help with alcoholism. In fact, the alcoholic person is more inclined to want help with problems that arise as a result of his drinking rather than with his drinking per se. To health professionals the person may present complaints of a physiologic nature, whereas the threat of divorce may lead him to a minister or social worker. When a client presents himself for help, it is important to recognize that even a tangential reference to drinking such as, "There's nothing wrong with my drinking, it is my wife who upsets me," may be an important clue to the presence of alcoholism. Other symptoms of the condition may become clear from the health history and physical examination, described in detail in Chapters 6 to 8. It is important for health professionals to recognize clues of alcoholism and to investigate and act on them in an appropriate manner.

Motivating the person toward acceptance of treatment

An opportune time to motivate the alcoholic person toward acceptance of treatment presents itself when the need for detoxification leads to hospitalization. A prolonged drinking bout, which eventually forces abstinence, often brings the alcoholic person to a health agency. At such times the client becomes acutely aware of physical deterioration; he feels the pain of self-loathing and humiliation, of isolation from family and friends, and that he is throwing away much of his unique and creative self.[34]

The nurse must take this opportunity to engage the client in a plan of treatment by confronting him in a nonjudgmental, serious manner with the symptoms of the disease process and by discussing treatment options with him. The client can be informed of available treatment modalities and helped to choose the one most suitable for him. He should be acquainted with the course alcoholism generally takes when alcoholic drinking continues.

To motivate the alcoholic person toward acceptance of treatment is the goal, and it is a difficult one to reach. The alcoholic person does not generally want to give up alcohol; all he wants is to be able to reduce his drinking. In spite of repeated failures to diminish alcohol intake, he continues to search for ways to achieve it. Even when he does begin to accept the premise that he needs help, it cannot be viewed as a lasting decision. Generally, as physical health improves, the motivation to enter treatment wanes. The nurse must be alert to subtle shifts in decisions and be creative in finding ways to enhance and maintain the alcoholic person's motivation to enter treatment. At such times, acquainting the client with a person who is recovering from alcoholism may help to reinforce a decision to enter treatment. Special interest shown by the nurse in the alcoholic client also is a potent factor in the reinforcement of the client's decision.

Once the alcoholic person agrees to enter a treatment program, the nurse assumes a much more active role than is usual in referring clients. Before transfer the client needs to be oriented to the prospective treatment program, preferably by a nurse or counselor of the treatment facility. Arrangements for transport to the agency must be secured, and the client should be accompanied by a family member or friend; if neither is available, the nurse may accompany the person. Once there, the client should be introduced to staff and clients of the treatment agency and left in the care of the counselor assigned to him.

Entering treatment is viewed by the alcoholic person as a means of robbing him of an essential ingredient of his life, the alcohol. He tends to seek any available means to escape this fate to the very end.

Enforced as opposed to voluntary treatment

Often the alcoholic person enters a treatment agency as a consequence of a court order because of legal infractions such as driving while intoxicated or having committed a negligent act while under the influence of alcohol. The person is forced to remain under treatment or risk incarceration. Although such severely imposed pressures do not always have a positive outcome, some persons benefit from the treatment experience, even under enforced conditions, and subsequently accept help voluntarily.

No matter what the circumstances are, it is important to use every opportunity to impress the client with the need for treatment. Although initially such attempts may fail, ultimately many persons realize that they cannot go on drinking and that they do need help.

DETOXIFICATION

Detoxification, although not a treatment for alcoholism in itself, is a vital first step in the recovery process. It is the period of abstinence from alcohol following a period of intoxication, during which the body rids itself of the alcohol. Although in nonaddicted persons this process tends to be benign, in the addicted individual it is not. When physical dependence on alcohol has developed, withdrawal symptoms appear in the form of tremors, hallucinations, seizures, and delirium tremens. The latter condition is a serious, life-threatening phenomenon, which is preventable.

Nature of the alcohol withdrawal syndrome

As described in Chapter 3, the alcohol withdrawal syndrome is a central nervous system response to the removal of alcohol from the body in the presence of physical dependence to the substance. Its most severe form, delirium tremens, is a life-threatening event, fatal to approximately 15% of the persons who are untreated, and must be viewed as an emergency.[33] If untreated, the initial symptoms of tremulousness, diaphoresis, weakness, and anorexia progress in a dose-time related sequence to nausea, vomiting, diarrhea, hypertension, hyperreflexia, fever, hallucinations, seizures, and finally delirium tremens. Although there are individual variations in dose and time thresholds, the occurrence of progressive symptoms can be estimated on the basis of the quantity of alcohol consumed per day and the length of time of its continuous intake. With such information, proper nursing management coupled with sedative therapy can be instituted to prevent the progression of withdrawal symptoms and to ameliorate existing ones.

Severe withdrawal reactions may occur in clients who, in addition to alcohol, have consumed other sedatives such as barbiturates or benzodiazepines. In the presence of multiple drug intake, the occurrence of symptoms after withdrawal of the drugs is likely to be delayed and prolonged. It is important to obtain laboratory information about the drugs present in the blood and to monitor the client's vital signs frequently. Symptoms likely to appear depend on factors such as types of drugs consumed, the extent of addiction, the client's nutritional status, fluid and electrolyte balance, and concurrent illnesses. When the combination of drugs consumed represents several central nervous system depressants, the danger of respiratory and cardiac depression is the greatest threat to the client's life.

Nursing management of the alcohol withdrawal syndrome

Nursing management during periods of detoxification can make the difference between safe recovery from the condition and an extremely stormy one. As mentioned earlier, major aims are to halt the progression of withdrawal symptoms and to ameliorate existing ones.

Initially, the nurse appraises the client for the presence of emergent conditions such as respiratory or cardiac embarrassment or excessive bleeding (p. 106). Next, a careful assessment of the client's recent drinking history is made. Information to be obtained includes length of the recent drinking bout, approximate quantity of alcohol consumed per day, time of last drink, nature of past withdrawal experiences, and presence of other chronic diseases or acute conditions. Based on the evaluation of this information, a plan of care is developed and management strategies are specified. Since the client may not be able to provide complete information, accompanying persons and previous hospital records are important sources to supplement the data. It is necessary not only to perform a careful appraisal of the client at the time of admission but to reevaluate him frequently for the development of complications.

Following are major areas in the continued evaluation and care of the client: (1) environment, (2) sedative replacement, (3) fluid and electrolyte replacement, and (4) nutrition.

Recovery from the withdrawal syndrome is enhanced in an atmosphere conducive to rest and relaxation. The client's room is kept free from disturbing stimuli. Noises, shadows, and sudden movements must be avoided. The room should be well lighted to avoid the elicitation of hallucinations and to facilitate orientation to the present. A quiet environment tends to decrease the incidence of withdrawal seizures, whereas extra stimuli such as sudden, shrill noises and jarring movements may elicit seizures in the agitated, hyperexcited client. A therapeutic milieu tends to decrease not only the severity of the withdrawal syndrome but also the amount of drug required for its management.

Most important are the attitudes displayed by persons caring for the alcoholic client and their abilities to convey support and acceptance. It has been said that the ultimate success or failure of treatment is related to the attitudes of treatment personnel. The nurse who is accepting of the alcoholic person and who understands what is happening during withdrawal is able to remain confident and is in a good position to provide necessary reassurance. As the nurse talks to the client in a quiet reassuring manner, orienting him to what is occurring, explaining the transitory nature of the unpleasant experiences, informing him of actions she is taking, anxiety and fear tend to decrease and to be replaced by feelings of relief and hope. In the absence of such support, or if the nurse transmits feelings of rejection, anxiety, or insecurity, the acutely anxious client in withdrawal may experience increased panic and the desire to escape.[12]

Sedative replacement therapy is known to stop progression of withdrawal symptoms effectively.[16] The principle of this therapy is to substitute a long-acting central nervous system depressant drug for the short-acting alcohol. Adequate sedation is aimed at producing a state of calm wakefulness. When this level of sedation is maintained for 1 or 2 days, it results in reduction of withdrawal symptoms and halts the progression to more serious ones. Drugs of choice include the benzodiazepines (minor tranquilizers) and barbiturates. Dosages must be carefully titrated against the client's weight and level of tolerance. The most sensitive indicator of adequate sedation is pulse rate, which should return to a rate within normal limits for the person. Decrease in anxiety and a state of restful calmness are additional signs of adequate levels of sedation. The dosage of the drug necessary to achieve this state of sedation is maintained for 24 to 48 hours and is then gradually reduced over a 2- to 3-day period until a zero level is reached.

Other important areas of care to be addressed during withdrawal are fluid and electrolyte balance and nutritional deficiencies. Fluid and electrolyte disturbances are common in the withdrawing patient; hypomagnesemia and hypokalemia are prevalent conditions. Although parenteral administration of magnesium sulfate and potassium may be indicated, oral administration of fruit juices and adequate dietary intake as soon as tolerated are the safest and most expeditious ways to correct for these disturbances.

The presence of multiple nutritional deficiencies is best counteracted with well-balanced meals. Short-term vitamin therapy may be indicated to replace deficiencies as well as to prevent further complications. For additional information on management during withdrawal, refer to "Diagnosis and Care of the Alcoholic Patient During Acute Episodes."[31]

Intoxication in the nonaddicted person usually simply leads to sleep. On awakening, the person generally is sober but may experience symptoms of "hangover" in the form of headache, nausea, vomiting, and dizziness. Recovery from the experience normally occurs without complications. No remedy, such as drinking black coffee or taking a cold shower, hastens the process of detoxification.

Settings for detoxification

Detoxification may occur without the help of health personnel or the support of professionals. The alcoholic person may simply taper off his drinking on his own. This form of detoxification is indeed common in persons with chronic alcoholism, but it is often an extremely painful process and not without danger. As was stated previously, the withdrawal phenomena may be life threatening.

Professional detoxification, as described before, occurs within a health care setting, under the care and supervision of nurses and physicians, and it involves the use of medication. This method of detoxification is referred to as the medical model.

In contrast is the social model of detoxification, which has received attention in recent years. It has been described as successful and safe for some patients.[24] Based on the philosophy that environmental manipulation is an effective alternative to chemotherapy, nonhospital personnel provide supervision and support to patients during withdrawal in a homelike environment that is warm, receptive, and free from excessive equipment and uniformed personnel.[24] Medications are generally not used. According to some authorities, paraprofessional personnel can be trained to detect potentially dangerous conditions and to refer persons with such conditions for appropriate care. Those with traumatic injuries and persons who are unable to walk are generally not admitted to social settings. Of those admitted, approximately 5% are referred to hospitals for further care.

Although social settings appear to provide acceptable conditions for some patients, the ultimate safety of this practice is not yet known. The course of withdrawal is not always predictable, and the mortality for persons inadequately treated remains high. On the other hand, high levels of safety with low mortality prevail when adequate professional treatment is provided.

LONG-TERM REHABILITATION

Ultimately, the long-term goal of alcoholism treatment is to help the person achieve an optimum level of health and to live the kind of life he considers acceptable. This goal often is painfully difficult and has been likened to climbing a steep icy hill. The alcoholic person goes up part of the way and then slips down a bit. By grabbing hold, he inches his way up slowly, a little further than he was before, until he hopefully and finally reaches the top.[5] Rehabilitation for the alcoholic person generally means a change in all ways of living. Finding new friends, another job, a new way of dealing with problems, and alternative means of managing stress all have to occur in the presence of physical discomfort engendered by the absence of the substance that formerly produced feelings of normality. Small wonder that often repeated efforts are necessary before a state of optimum health and rehabilitation is reached.

Factors related to successful treatment

Although rehabilitation from alcoholism is difficult, 30% to 40% of persons presenting themselves for treatment are said to achieve this goal.[25] In comparison with other chronic illnesses, alcoholism is regarded as a highly treatable condition.

The enhancement of effective treatment has remained a major concern of health professionals. Efforts, however, have been hampered partly by conflicting reports of what characteristics tend to relate to success in treatment. For instance, neither the kind of treatment modality nor the length of treatment efforts has provided clear indications of relationship to recovery. In fact, some studies have shown rates of recovery for persons in control groups (those receiving no treatment) to be very similar to persons in treatment groups.[10] Other researchers using different treatment modalities have found that desirable outcomes were related to client characteristics of social stability, intellectual superiority, psychological intactness, and the presence of motivation.[15] Characteristics of this type are indicators of success in almost any kind of intervention and therefore provide little guidance for treatment of the vast number of persons who do not have this constellation of characteristics. At present, success of treatment designed to rehabilitate the alcoholic person appears to be primarily related to the degree to which an individualized approach to the client's problems is used.

Two practices that appear to enhance the outcome of treatment are concurrent family therapy and provision for continuation of care. The recognition that all members of an alcoholic person's family tend to develop sociopsychological problems and that their problems tend to be interdependent has led treatment personnel to focus on family therapy as an approach to alcoholism rehabilitation. When used, family therapy indeed appears to increase the likelihood of success in rehabilitation of alcoholic persons.

It has long been recognized that changes in the behavior of one family member are accompanied by corresponding changes in the family as a whole. In the process of developing alcoholism, the alcoholic member increasingly is unable to carry out expected family roles, causing the family unit to cease to function smoothly. In the ensuing turmoil, conflicts are engendered among all family members and usually result in multiple interpersonal and intrapersonal problems. Eventually a new level of smooth family functioning is reached, generally without the alcoholic person. Disturbances tend to recur at times when the alcoholic member attempts to reenter the family unit, often subsequent to treatment experiences.

Family therapy aims to deal with existing disturbances and to prevent others. By involving the entire family unit in a therapeutic endeavor, major goals are the improvement of communications, the reestablishment of trust relationships, and the realignment of family responsibilities. An important component of the process is to teach the entire family about the nature of alcoholism. As all family members become informed about it and as they mutually participate in the recovery processes, changes in the home environment and the family structure ensue and contribute to a more lasting recovery of the alcoholic person.

Follow-up care after a period of treatment provides a link that strengthens rehabilitation efforts. The alcoholic person needs, for some time to come, support for and reinforcement of the values inherent in life without alcohol, and he often needs assistance with emerging problems. Alcoholics Anonymous has consistently provided such support for its members by nature of its practices. Other treatment agencies have also recognized the importance of continued group support as an adjunct to therapy. Posttreatment or follow-up programs take the form of regularly scheduled group meetings or as telephone contact made with clients at regular intervals. Alcoholics Anonymous and alcoholism outpatient services are often used as systems of continued care, and occasionally clients discharged from treatment organize their own posttherapy.

In recent years halfway houses for persons recovering from alcoholism have increased in some communities. Defined as "transitional places of indefinite residence of a community of persons who live together under the rule and discipline of abstinence from alcohol and other drugs,"[16] they came into being to offer support to the alcoholic person while he is learning to become self-sufficient. Through intimate association with other persons seeking similar goals, problems encountered in maintaining abstinence, in assuming job responsibilities, and in communicating with other people are confronted in group meetings. Generally, the alcoholic person is free to become employed while living at the halfway house as long as he adheres to established resident rules. He generally also determines the length of his stay at this facility himself. For a certain group of alcoholic people, living in a halfway house prior to independent living provides the added support needed to secure lasting rehabilitation.

Major treatment modalities

A variety of treatment approaches and techniques have been developed and used to deal with alcoholism. As mentioned earlier, research has not yet demonstrated convincingly that any one approach works better with specific groups of people than any other. Major approaches in current use include Alcoholics Anonymous, counseling, behavioral approaches, and deterrent agents.

Alcoholics Anonymous

Alcoholics Anonymous (AA) is a major organization for the treatment of alcoholism that is readily available in virtually every community in the United States. It was founded in 1935 in Akron, Ohio, by two alcoholic men, Bill Wilson, a stockbroker, and Dr. Bob Smith, a physician. These two men discovered that they could stay sober through mutual support, helping one another, not as a professional helper to a patient but as one peer to another sharing their common experiences with alcoholism.[9] As part of their recovery program, they began working with other alcoholic persons, who, in turn, worked with still others. Gradually small groups of sober alcoholics were meeting in several cities throughout the United States. From its humble beginnings in Ohio, Alcoholics Anonymous grew rapidly over a four-decade span into a successful worldwide self-help movement for the treatment of alcoholism. Largely through its successful efforts, alcoholism is no longer viewed as a hopeless condition but rather as a treatable illness from which many alcoholic persons can recover. In addition, Alcoholics Anonymous has become the model for other successful self-help groups such as Overeaters Anonymous and Parents Anonymous.

Alcoholics Anonymous is governed at the national level by the General Service Board, composed of both alcoholic and nonalcoholic persons who deal with the organization's business and financial concerns. Locally, each group is self-supporting with expenses, such as rent for a meeting place and refreshments, met by passing the hat at meetings. As a rule, meetings take place in public buildings, often a church, where rent is either free or nominal in amount. There are no fees or dues for membership, making it possible for anyone, regardless of economic status, to participate. The only requirement for membership is a desire on the part of the alcoholic person to stop drinking.

In large metropolitan areas, simultaneous group meetings take place in several locations at almost every hour throughout the day and evening. Attendance ranges from a few people to as many as a hundred. There are AA groups composed primarily of homogeneous populations such as youth, women, homosexuals, and professional persons. There are heterogeneous groups with members derived from both sexes, various socioeconomic strata, and different age groups. Some groups are more energetic, insightful, successful, and serious than others. If one particular AA group fails to meet the individual needs of an alcoholic person, another group functioning at another, often nearby, location may prove to be more appealing and helpful.

Meetings are either open or closed. Open meetings may be attended by any interested person; closed meetings are conducted for alcoholic persons only. Meetings, as a rule, follow a fairly regular format with a chairperson opening the meeting with a moment of silence, and then the Serenity Prayer is recited by everyone: "God grant me the serenity to accept the things I cannot change, the courage to change the things I can, and the wisdom to know the difference."

After the prayer the purpose of AA is presented. A statement is read that AA is a fellowship of men and women who share their experience, strength, and hope with one another to solve their similar problem and help others recover from alcoholism. AA's sole purpose is to help individual members stay sober, and they, in turn, help other alcoholic persons to achieve sobriety. The Twelve Steps that embody the philosophy of AA and provide specific guidelines on how to attain and maintain sobriety are then read. In this series of steps, members admit they are powerless over alcohol, develop complete reliance on a Power greater than themselves, become involved in honest self-analysis and catharsis, make restitution to people they have harmed, and give of themselves to other persons with alcoholism without expectation of reward.

At some meetings the reading of the Twelve Steps is followed by the Twelve Traditions. The latter are statements of policy concerning how AA operates as an organization. The traditions stress factors such as the autonomy of each group, the nonprofessional nature of AA, the fact that AA does not engage in any controversy or express any opinion on outside issues, and the importance of anonymity to remind members to place principles above personalitites. In keeping with the tradition of anonymity, last names of members are not used.

A member of the group then gives a short talk on an alcohol-related subject such as reiterating one of the Twelve Steps and discussing any difficulties and successes the person has experienced in achieving the step. Other times the member may read a passage from the book entitled *Alcoholics Anonymous*,[1] often referred to as the "big book." This book was first printed in 1939 and since then has been reprinted many times. It contains the story of how many thousands of men and women have recovered from alcoholism through AA. Another book the speaker may choose to quote is *The AA Way of Life* by Bill Wilson, one of the co-founders of AA. Every person is given an opportunity to talk during the open discussion period that follows the reading. For example, a person might relate how his experience with alcoholism coincides with or differs from those of other members. When the attendance is large, members often form small groups for the discussion period. The session closes with the Lord's Prayer.

After the session there is a good deal of social interaction among members, as they drink coffee, eat refreshments, and informally share their experiences. During both the formal and informal exchanges, members learn what AA believes about alcoholism. In AA it is generally accepted that alcoholism is an illness and that total abstinence is the only successful way by which alcoholism can be arrested. AA does not endorse controlled drinking research and teaches that an alcoholic person can never safely return to social drinking. AA emphasizes that sobriety is achieved by not drinking one day at a time. Guilt about one's past is alleviated and excess anxiety about the future is curtailed by focusing on the present.

A number of important concepts operate in AA to make it an effective means of therapy for many alcoholic people. Members interact in an atmosphere of mutual acceptance and support. Participation is by choice. Those who do not find AA helpful tend to withdraw, leaving persons who are achieving success to serve as role models for new members. The pressure to change drinking behavior and the way to attain and maintain sobriety are provided by peers with similar histories and goals. As members successfully learn abstinent behavior, their self-esteem increases and they gradually become able to help newcomers to AA in the way that they have been helped. The latter refers to the "helper therapy" principle whereby the person providing assistance derives greater benefits than those to whom the help is being offered. Group acceptance, use of successful role models, peer pressure, and helping oneself through helping others are a few of the concepts operative in AA and in other self-help organizations.

Nurses need to be fully and accurately informed about AA as an important and necessary treatment resource on the health care continuum so that they can make use of AA as a referral source for alcoholic clients. At a minimum, every alcoholic person needs to know about AA at least to the point where he can make an informed decision regarding its personal effectiveness for him. Some persons will find in AA all they need to know to recover from alcoholism, others will use it as supplemental to other forms of help, whereas still others will choose means entirely separate from AA to achieve recovery status.

Counseling

Individual counseling is used in most clinical settings as part or all of the treatment of alcoholic persons. It is often used in combination with other modalities including group therapy, drug therapy such as disulfiram (Antabuse), and Alcoholics Anonymous.

In the course of individual counseling, a helping person offers a client a structured, constructive, interpersonal relationship in which brief encounters between the counselor and client occur over a period of weeks, months, or years. As a result of involvement in counseling, the client can expect to develop increased self-understanding and improved day-to-day functioning—changes that will enable him to live in a more positive and productive way. The length of counseling varies, and it is a purposeful, goal-directed relationship, factors that need to be well understood by the participants.

Generally speaking, those persons most successful in their efforts to counsel alcoholic clients focus on current reality, active development of a working treatment relationship, environmental manipulation, and strengthening ego assets. Counselors who tend to be passive in developing a therapeutic alliance and who are oriented toward investigation and interpretation of inner experiences are less successful in their efforts with alcoholic clients.[4]

Alcoholism counselors, in general, possess varied professional backgrounds and may include nurses with specialized knowledge and skill in both counseling and alcoholism. Nurses may counsel alcoholic clients, for example, as a part of their employment in an alcoholism section of an outpatient community mental health center, a residential treatment program for alcoholism, or in a private practice setting. Whatever the counselor's background, alcoholic clients need exceptionally competent counselors who are warm, kind, and nonjudgmental yet able to set limits firmly. The counselor needs to be able to acknowledge mistakes forthrightly and to share feelings nondefensively that arise during counseling.

The counseling relationship can be described as having three phases: initial, middle, and final. Each phase is fairly distinct, although overlapping in nature with the others. The phases will be discussed, highlighting several commonly occurring aspects that need to be dealt with when counseling alcoholic clients. The subject of counseling alcoholic clients is covered comprehensively elsewhere.[40] Although the emphasis here is on individual counseling, it can be assumed that similar aspects would need to be included whether the modality instituted is individual, group, or family therapy.

Initial phase. As in all counseling relationships, one of the first tasks with an alcoholic client is to outline a treatment plan, sometimes referred to as a contract. The contract involves the establishment of a regularly scheduled time of meeting, some consideration of the proposed length of counseling, fees, the handling of changes in appointments and cancelled hours, a discussion of the goals of treatment, and an explanation of the way the nurse works to help achieve the goals.

A basic step in setting counseling goals consists of the nurse asking the client some form of the question: "What do you expect to get out of counseling?" and "How will you achieve your expectations?" The client's initial responses are often general in nature, such as "I have no self-confidence," or "I must stop drinking," or "I want my children back." Additional steps in discussing goals involve further questions by the nurse to help the client specify attainable expectations and to differentiate short- and long-term goals.

When the client arrives at a set of reasonably realistic goals, the nurse summarizes them and indicates if and how the goals might be achieved in counseling. Goals are constantly under review and changing. They are not to be inflexibly pursued, but they do form a framework around which counseling can proceed. One alcoholic man, after successfully determining a set of initial goals for the counseling sessions, stated, "When I know what course I'm taking, I can usually make the grade."

Goals that apply to drinking or not drinking need to be specifically defined, since alcoholism is often the major life problem for which alcoholic persons seek help. The nurse's viewpoint on this essential issue needs to be clear. The nurse counselor may select one of several positions, depending on her own beliefs about alcoholism and on the needs of individual clients. The most common position is that the client must achieve lifelong abstinence as soon as possible. A variant of this position involves taking no stand on lifelong abstinence but demanding abstinence during the course of counseling. Espousal of abstinence indicates a belief that alcoholism is a disease accompanied by loss of control over alcohol intake.[4]

A position at the other end of the spectrum is also possible. This involves taking a neutral viewpoint on the issue of drinking and assuming the client is not drinking or at least not in ways that deleteriously affect the course of treatment. With this view the nurse sees excessive drinking as a symptom of an underlying emotional disturbance. Counseling follows fairly traditional notions that self-understanding of conflicts giving rise to the symptom will result in symptom removal and direct attacks on the symptom will prove valueless.[4]

A fairly closely allied position is that of remaining neutral about the issue of eventual drinking but explicitly prohibiting drinking prior to or during counseling sessions. Nurses adhering to this position believe that meaningful emotional experiences cannot occur when the client's state of consciousness has been altered by a drug.[4]

Another option, more recently defined, is one in which the nurse explicitly discusses with selected clients the goal of moderating alcohol intake rather than achieving abstinence. Youthful clients without advanced physical sequelae of alcoholism, for example, may outrightly reject an abstinence goal but may adjust reasonably well to moderating the amount and frequency of drinking. Nurses who offer this option believe that excessive drinking is essentially a learned phenomenon. Counseling would include efforts such as reducing stress in the client's life to make alcohol less important and encouraging peer relationships with persons who use alcohol in socially accepted ways.

The problem with any of these positions is that at some point in the course of counseling the alcoholic client is likely to appear for a session in an inebriated state. The question, then, for the nurse becomes one of how to deal with drunkenness if it occurs in a counseling session. Although there are no pat answers to this question, nurses have an obligation to be thoroughly familiar with the client's drinking history. The nurse quickly assesses whether the intoxicated client needs detoxification in an inpatient facility or if he primarily needs assistance to reach a place safely where he can sleep off the effects of intoxication. Some nurses assume drunkenness is a form of communication, and if the client is not disruptive or too sedated, they make use of the counseling session to define what the person is saying by his behavior.

Removing alcohol from the alcoholic person's life is often a painful, complex process. Creating and adjusting to a life without alcohol is an ordeal and involves recognizing all that alcohol has done for the person. When the client reaches the point of giving up alcohol, the question is, "What will take its place?" Something new and constructive must be added to fill the void, and clients must work diligently to discover what can adequately replace alcohol in their lives.

Another important aspect of the initial stage involves working with the client's defenses, which often include some degree of denial. The alcoholic client is likely to doubt the severity of his condition and spends an extraordinary amount of time and energy trying to convince himself and others that drinking poses no real difficulties for him. The client needs help to look at his doubt without debate or argument. Exploring what happens when a drinking bout occurs is often useful. Can the client stop drinking whenever he chooses to? What are the consequences of his drinking? Does he ultimately behave in ways that humiliate himself and others? Do drinking episodes increasingly alienate him from others? The goal of this exploration is to enable the client to accept, and say in his own words, exactly how drinking is a disruptive force in his life. It is less important that he accept the label of "alcoholic," which carries a stigma for many people.[37]

A final aspect of the initial phase involves encouraging the client to share the work of counseling. It is essential from the beginning to convey to the client that he must work in therapy. Frequently, the client will become "emotionally flabby," that is, change or refuse to pursue a subject, just when he needs to stay with an idea or when he is on the verge of making some real progress.[29] At the same time the nurse may inadvertently play into this tendency. The following example illustrates these points. The interaction takes place between a nurse counselor and an alcoholic client in the second counseling session. In this episode they have been discussing possible goals for counseling and, specifically, whether the client does or does not have control over his drinking.

Nurse: I'm hearing two ideas from you. One is that you have control over your drinking. You plan for it so you have control over it. I also hear you saying that sometimes even when you plan to limit your drinking, you don't—you go out and get drunk. Those are two opposite things that happen to you. Is that correct?

Client: I don't know, I'm so completely confused that I don't really know.

Nurse: It seems you have experienced both of those things. You have good evidence for both of the things you said, and you're saying both at the same time. I think that would be an important issue for us to look at, because that may be confusing you.

Client: Could be. You probably think I'm really a weird person. I'm so confused about . . . don't ask me what I'm confused about, I don't know what I'm confused about . . . I'm just confused . . .

Nurse: That's understandable, you're trying to think about whether you can control your drinking and you come up with two different explanations as to what happens when you drink. Both are reasonable. I think that's confusing.

In this example the client expresses an unwillingness to think, and so the nurse attempts to think for him. At the same time there is danger that the client is taken "off the hook" if given too much understanding. Instead, the nurse needs to convey to the client that it is possible for him to clarify his confusion, but it requires thought and a willingness to work. The client who repeatedly says "I don't know" or similar phrases is discounting his ability to solve problems. Alcoholic clients often have developed a habit of obliterating reality with alcohol rather than puzzling it out with reasoned thought. A major task of counseling, permeating all phases of the relationship, is to encourage the client's active involvement in the development and use of problem-solving and decision-making skills.

Middle phase. In the middle phase of counseling it is important to study the reasons why the person drinks. What is the power of the addiction? What effects is the person seeking from alcohol? This is different from looking for reasons why a person has alcoholism. The former focuses on the here and now rather than searching into one's past. For example, when a drinking episode occurs, it is helpful to look in depth at the following: What led up to it, the actual drinking behavior, and what happened as a result of the drinking? Collecting data from several drinking episodes allows the nurse and client to compare what occurred and to determine more clearly what the client needs to do to change his behavior.

The following account quotes the same client cited earlier as he describes what led to a particular drinking episode. He is working on the question of whether he usually planned to get drunk or whether drunkenness simply happened without forethought on his part.

Client: I remember now. The other day I was in town. I went into a bar at 10 AM. I was looking for somebody. I met an old friend and I sat there and had a drink with him. As a matter of fact, I had several drinks with him. Then I went next door to the tavern to see if my friend was there—she wasn't. I saw a lady there I knew, so I sat with her and talked with her and had a couple of beers. Then, *all of a sudden* something went click. I said it's a nice day. I'm going to get drunk! I didn't walk in there to get drunk, I had just walked in there *to see if my old lady was there*, and I had a couple and then I went over there and had a couple more. I just said the heck with it and decided to get drunk. That's happened quite a few times.

Frequently, as in this example, in studying the client's accounts it becomes clearer how he fails to recognize feelings aroused in interpersonal transactions and to deal with these feelings constructively. Instead, the client automatically drinks. In discussing this episode with the nurse, the client saw in retrospect that he was expecting to find his "old lady" in the first bar and that failure to do so caused him to feel angry. Since anger was discomforting to him, he attempted to erase the pain through habitual drinking. Drinking in response to uncomfortable intrapersonal and interpersonal situations, such as those involving anger, is common among alcoholic persons,[20] and often leads to a relapse.

In counseling, the client learns that feelings are useful in alerting one to the fact that something is personally troublesome. Feelings can be recognized by determining where in one's body discomfort or tenseness is felt. Many people, for example, get "knots" in the stomach when they experience extreme feelings. The knots in the stomach become the signal that something is awry. The next step is for the client to name the feeling, whether it be anger, fear, sadness, or some other feeling and then to use recognition of the feeling as a springboard for involvement in problem-solving activity. The nurse helps by asking the client questions such as, "Where in your body do you feel discomfort?" "name the feeling," "put the feeling into words," or "talk about the feeling." Rather than drinking, the person learns to subject disquieting feelings to instant analysis. In so doing, the client postpones relief of discomfort and in the process explores what is happening. As he accomplishes this, he is buying time to develop reasoned thought regarding alternative responses to life situations. Ultimately, the client learns that feelings are helpful in identifying that problems exist, but they are not helpful in solving problems. Thinking is the most essential component in solving problems and in making behavioral changes.[6]

Homework assignments designed to extend the work of counseling into the client's daily life are often useful. One such assignment involves practicing self-analysis in interactions occurring outside the counseling sessions. With time and guided effort the alcoholic person learns increasingly to turn to alternative solutions, rather than drinking, in response to painful emotion. He learns to unwind and to be socially at ease without alcohol. In spite of the fact that society stacks the deck in favor of drinking by making it seem acceptable and readily available, ultimately, many alcoholic clients choose to deal with life without alcohol. This calls for a particularly mature adjustment to life, one that the average, nonaddicted person is not called on to make.

In the course of counseling, the abstinent alcoholic client will sometimes experience a resurgence of behavior typical of his drinking days. This is sometimes referred to as "dry drunk," a term describing the state of the alcoholic person who is uncomfortable when not drinking.[30] An outstanding characteristic of the "dry drunk" is overreaction. The client temporarily develops grandiose behavior, exaggerating his importance at the expense of others, makes highly judgmental value statements about himself and others, and is tensely impatient. The client may be finding it extremely difficult to accept what he is learning about himself in his sober state, and his behavior may be an effort to preserve his self-esteem. It is a time for the counselor to help him understand what is happening, to tolerate the discomfort, and to develop increased self-discipline. With these efforts the symptoms of "dry drunk" are likely to subside in a matter of several days without the client's resorting to past patterns of drinking to relieve emotional discomfort.

Final phase. The final phase of counseling is an extremely important part of therapy. For alcoholic clients termination sometimes occurs too abruptly, such as when negative feelings erupt on the part of the client without his making constructive efforts to resolve them. On the other hand, termination is sometimes unnecessarily delayed because the client becomes comfortable in the counseling relationship and does not wish to have this security disrupted. In such instances the counselor must guard against allowing the client to make counseling a permanent way of life.

From the beginning of counseling, eventual termination is the goal, and the circumscribed nature of therapy needs to be made clear to the client. Establishing that an alcoholic client is ready for termination requires that satisfactory answers to a number of questions be obtained, such as the following:

Has the client achieved significant progress in regard to stated counseling goals?

Can he communicate nondefensively most of the time?

Can he choose a reaction, handling the activities and demands of daily life without recourse to alcohol?

To what extent is he involved in a well-rounded life, using a number of external resources such as hobbies, new friends, and constructive outlets for energy, such as sports?

Is the client making use of more of his internal resources with consistent, constructive involvement in work and in meaningful interpersonal relations?

In the final analysis, it is not whether or not the client has problems but, rather, how he reacts to and handles them.

Since ending a relationship is not a simple procedure, the feelings activated by termination, most notably fear and anger, need to be experienced slowly. A period of several weeks or months usually provides ample time for the client to recognize and work through emotions aroused by separation.

The final sessions are also a time to take stock of accomplishments, including progress toward stated goals. They are a time to underscore the strengths that the client possesses and to determine areas where continued growth may be indicated. The client needs to realize that the development of increased self-understanding and achievement of more fulfilling functioning is a lifelong process and counseling is only a beginning to that end.

Behavioral approaches

Behavioral scientists propose that, for a segment of the alcoholic population, alcoholism is an acquired behavior maintained by known mechanisms of learning and that for these persons it can be modified and perhaps eliminated by applying techniques derived from principles of learning.[21] Behaviorists place emphasis on the assessment of antecedent and consequent events related to excessive drinking and on the use of social learning techniques that can serve as alternatives to drinking.

A popular behavioral position has been that alcohol reduces stress and anxiety and that alcoholics have learned to use alcohol in an attempt to reduce unpleasant emotions. On this basis therapeutic approaches employed as alternatives to alcohol use have been those which reduce stress and tension. To alter tension and subsequent drinking, the alcoholic person is taught techniques such as social and self-management skills, assertive behavior, and relaxation methods such as meditation, muscular relaxation, and biofeedback.

Assertiveness in particular has been useful to the alcoholic person who is learning to counteract social pressures to drink and to communicate effectively without experiencing anxiety. Assertive behavior means that the individual can express personal rights and feelings in a socially acceptable fashion and can stand up for himself without generating undue anxiety.[22] The alcoholic person has been said to be lacking in assertive skills. When interpersonal situations require assertive behavior and the person does not possess assertive skills, tension tends to be generated. To overcome unpleasant feelings of tension, the alcoholic person drinks. With proficiency in assertiveness skills, the alcoholic person becomes more competent in interpersonal communications and feels better about himself. It is hypothesized that avoidance of tension and improvement in the concept of self tend to reduce the need for alcohol intake. Further studies are necessary to validate this hypothesis.

Biofeedback is a technique that is used to relax and desensitize a person to high levels of anxiety. It involves the use of physiologic signals for the self-regulation of specific physiologic processes and has been helpful for alcoholic persons in combating anxiety and tension reactions. As the alcoholic person learns to control physiologic processes such as increasing the temperature in his hands, reducing muscle tension levels, and increasing the percentage of alpha rhythms, he begins to realize that he has the power to make changes within himself and a sense of self-mastery ensues. With this new knowledge some alcoholic persons have obtained a high degree of freedom from alcohol.[14]

The regular practice of meditation, a state of relaxation characterized by decreases in oxygen consumption, carbon dioxide elimination, and lowered respiratory rate, has been found to result in a significant decrease in alcohol consumption by nonalcoholic individuals. Its effects on persons with alcoholism, however, are not yet known.[2]

Another approach in the realm of behavioral therapy is physical exercise. When used with alcoholic persons, exercise improved their general state of health as well as self-esteem and tended to reduce alcoholic drinking.[13]

An early behavioral approach, pioneered in a Seattle hospital, is an application of Pavlov's classic conditioning model to the treatment of alcoholism.[19] With the use of aversive stimuli of an emetic or electric shock, a negative association with the sight, smell, and taste of alcohol is created. Any consideration of drinking thereafter reflexly evokes nausea or pain, and the idea of drinking is rejected. Since the conditioned reflex weakens with time, repeated periodic treatments are necessary to maintain the aversive response. The major gain from this form of treatment is that it reduces the craving for alcoholic drinking, permitting the alcoholic person to reorder his life. Although no controlled studies have been reported, conditioning has resulted in high abstinence rates for at least two years for some persons.

Deterrent agents

Numerous pharmacologic agents have been used and tested in an effort to deter the consumption of alcohol. Drugs have been used to counteract anxiety and depression related to alcohol intake, to set up aversive responses to alcohol, and to interfere with alcohol consumption.

Antianxiety and antidepressant drugs. Chlordiazepoxide (Librium) and diazepam (Valium) are two drugs of the benzodiazepine group that have been studied in connection with their long-term effectiveness in relieving anxiety and depression in alcoholic persons. Neither drug has been shown to bring about dramatic changes in dysphoria of patients or in long-term changes in drinking behavior. Since both resemble alcohol in their psychologic and physiologic effects on the person, the likelihood exists that the client may develop physical dependence on the drugs. Although these drugs are safe and effective in treating withdrawal symptoms, thus far it appears that they do not have a valid place in the long-term treatment of alcoholism.

A drug that appears to have some promise in reducing drinking episodes is lithium carbonate. It has been used in the treatment of manic depressive disorders. Observations of decreased drinking episodes in persons treated with lithium led to a study that compared chronic alcoholics and nonpsychotic depressed persons receiving lithium with a control group receiving placebos. It was found that those using lithium were significantly less likely to have disabling drinking episodes.[17] Before taking a stand on its ultimate usefulness in the treatment of alcoholism, further evidence of this drug's effectiveness must be obtained.

Aversive agents. As was mentioned earlier, aversive agents are used to generate an association of unpleasant stimuli (nausea, vomiting, paralysis of muscles) with the consumption of alcoholic beverages. Emetine and apomorphine, drugs that produce vomiting, have been used to set up an aversion to the sight, smell, and taste of alcohol. Succinylcholine, a drug that causes brief, overall paralysis of muscles, has been used to create an aversion reflex. It is a potentially dangerous agent, and its use in alcoholism treatment has been largely abandoned.

Drugs interfering with alcohol consumption. A drug that is widely used in long-term treatment of alcoholism and is an effective adjunct to therapy is disulfiram (Antabuse). This drug has little or no effect on the person in the absence of alcohol ingestion. When alcohol is consumed while disulfiram is in the body, the metabolism of alcohol is blocked, and an accumulation of acetaldehyde, a toxic metabolic product of alcohol, ensues. The symptoms of such an accumulation, in order of appearance, are flushing, sweating, palpitations, dyspnea, hyperventilation, tachycardia, hypotension, nausea, and vomiting. The reaction is dose dependent, but only minimal amounts of alcohol and disulfiram are sufficient to produce the reaction.[7] Although extremely unpleasant and often frightening to the person, the symptoms generally subside and the person completely recovers. Disulfiram is a long-acting drug and may continue to cause reactions for days after its ingestion has been stopped, particularly in persons with heart disease.

In general, disulfiram is useful for persons who are motivated to recover. Although it does not provide a cure, it aids in keeping the person from impulsive drinking, thus providing time during which the individual can learn to manage life without the use of alcohol. Since the taking of the drug is under the person's control, it provides him with a sense of power over his destiny, increasing confidence and self-esteem. Disulfiram is most useful as an adjunct to other therapeutic interventions.

One group of alcoholic clients who do less well with disulfiram therapy than others are those who are depressed. The basis for this occurrence is not known. In one study depression acted as a specific negative prognostic factor in disulfiram therapy.[15]

When taking disulfiram, the person must be told of foods and compounds that are likely to contain alcohol. He must avoid gourmet dinners, for instance, which may include foods prepared with wines, and medications such as cough syrups that often contain alcohol. It is also advisable for him to wear a bracelet which indicates that "this person is taking disulfiram."

Disulfiram subcutaneous implants have been developed and used with varying success. Persons with implants tended to refrain from drinking for longer periods than did persons in a control group with whom they were compared.[38] Problems resulting from this method were unpredictable, however, and they included loss of effectiveness in inducing the typical disulfiram-alcohol reaction and infections at sites of implantation.

A drug used primarily in England and Canada with disulfiram-like actions is citrated calcium cyanamide. Another deterrent agent, metronidazole, has also been used; it is a chemical that initially appeared to induce a distaste to alcohol. Studies, however, showed only minimal effectiveness of this drug.[7]

Alcoholism services

In the past several years the number and kind of alcoholism services have proliferated so that in most major communities a range of treatment settings for rehabilitation of alcoholic persons is available. These include community alcohol centers, alcohol inpatient treatment facilities, alcohol outpatient clinics, and groups of Alcoholics Anonymous. Multiple treatment approaches are used, and varying successes with clients have been recorded in most of these settings with all of them.

Community alcohol centers

Community alcohol centers, supported by federal, state, and local funds, have been a major resource in the rehabilitation of alcoholic persons. Initially they were established to provide information about alcoholism to the community to aid in the identification of alcoholic persons and to act as a central resource for referral to other agencies; now they generally also have a treatment dimension. Group, individual, and family counseling is provided in addition to services related to the identification of the alcohol problem, education about alcoholism, and referral to other treatment agencies. The clientele are derived from referrals made by health professionals, family members, friends, and self-referrals. In addition, a large proportion of clients are court referred.

Personnel of the agency generally include some health professionals, such as social workers and nurses, but consist primarily of counselors who are themselves recovered alcoholic persons. Seeking help from a community alcoholism center may be the alcoholic person's first attempt to deal with alcoholism, and the quality of interaction with agency personnel may be critical to the client's subsequent behavior. After the nature of problems has been evaluated, a referral to a suitable agency may be made or the person may be engaged in a counseling relationship provided by the agency. The role of nurses in a community alcohol center depends on their professional preparation. To provide alcohol education, to counsel clients, and to make assessments and referrals are all within the purview of nursing and are functions variably assumed by nurses in community alcohol centers.

The nurse is in a strategic position to refer persons with alcohol problems to a community alcohol center for evaluation, information, and treatment. It is a useful agency not only for the alcoholic person but also for family members and other concerned persons. Here the nature of the alcohol problem is assessed and the many questions that have occurred to family members and to the alcoholic person are freely discussed.

Systematic evaluations of the effectiveness of community alcohol centers are sparse. Studies have shown that these agencies may serve a pivotal function in terms of coordinating and catalyzing rehabilitation efforts.[8]

Alcohol inpatient treatment facilities

The three major types of inpatient facilities for the treatment of alcoholic persons are mental hospitals, general hospitals, and specialty alcoholism treatment facilities. Historically, state mental hospitals have provided treatment for alcoholism to large numbers of persons. As many as 40% of all men admitted to mental hospitals have a diagnosis of alcoholism, and approximately 10% of state mental hospitals have special alcoholism wards, which provide care and treatment for alcoholic persons.[26] Group psychotherapy, didactic lectures, discussions, and Alcoholics Anonymous meetings have been the treatment approaches most frequently used in these settings. Concepts of "therapeutic community" and "milieu therapy" are employed, emphasizing the use of the client's total daily experience as an effort to improve his functioning. Mental hospitals in the past have not involved family members in treatment efforts, and aftercare services have been lacking. Improvements are being made, leading to more effective treatment of clients.

The provision of alcoholism treatment services within general hospitals is a relatively recent occurrence. Promoted by the American Hospital Association, general hospitals increasingly provide treatment and care to alcoholic clients either in specialty wards or as an integral part of other major services.

For some time the development of services for alcoholic clients within general hospitals has been hampered, partly because health professionals tended to ignore the problem of alcoholism while providing care and treatment for alcohol-related diseases. Hospitalization for conditions such as withdrawal, hepatic disease, or gastrointestinal bleeding usually represent a crisis in the life of an alcoholic person and offer an important opportunity to engage the client in treatment for alcoholism. Yet in many instances the client has been discharged after the alcohol-related condition has been treated, and no attempt has been made to deal with the alcoholism. As a consequence, the revolving-door syndrome develops. The alcoholic person returns repeatedly for treatment of related conditions, simply because the source of the problem has remained unchanged. This situation is beginning to change as more health professionals become knowledgeable about alcoholism and general hospitals recognize alcoholism as a treatable condition.

When a general hospital has a special unit for the treatment of alcoholic persons, it may be organized in the pattern of other hospital units, with a nurse as administrator, or it may be formed with counseling services as the central component of the unit, often with the head counselor as unit manager. In either organizational pattern the unit teams typically consist of both health professionals (physicians, nurses, aides) and alcoholism counselors (psychologists, social workers, recovering alcoholics with training in counseling).

Treatment provided to alcoholic clients is comprehensive, including both health services for acute and chronic conditions and treatment for alcoholism. In general, treatment for alcoholism consists of group and individual counseling, behavior modification, and education. Alcoholics Anonymous is usually an integral part of therapy, and increasingly, family therapy and follow-up care are part of the overall treatment plan.

The provision of services for alcoholic clients within general hospitals moves the care of alcoholic persons into the mainstream of the nation's social and health care delivery system, a direction promoted by federal agencies. In these settings the potential for comprehensive care of all existing health problems, including alcoholism, is enhanced, and as the level of care of alcoholic persons improves, so does their prognosis for rehabilitation.[34]

In general, it can be said that alcoholic persons who experience symptoms that are primarily related to illnesses resulting from alcoholism (gastritis, pancreatitis, hepatitis) tend to present themselves for treatment to health care professionals and appear in health care agencies such as clinics or hospitals. Following treatment of acute conditions, referral to alcoholism treatment agencies may ensue. Alcoholic persons without serious physical complications tend to present themselves or are referred directly to alcoholism treatment agencies.

A fundamental kind of inpatient service for alcoholic persons is provided by free-standing agencies specializing in treatment for alcoholism. Specialty alcoholism care units have proliferated in the past decade. They often are nonprofit organizations, conducting treatment programs ranging in length from 3 to 6 weeks. The orientation tends to be one of involving the person in bringing about changes in personal life-style. Group and individual therapy, as well as approaches geared toward learning new ways of behavior, providing didactic information about alcoholism, and linking the person to Alcoholics Anonymous are some of the treatment modalities offered.

Although most specialty care units offer a variety of treatment modalities, some employ only specialty methods. One modality is "aversion conditioning," which is used as major therapy in some well-known institutions. The personnel comprise a large counseling staff and a selected number of health professionals. The counseling staff typically consist of persons who are recovered alcoholics and who have had varying degrees of educational preparation in alcoholism counseling. These persons are dedicated to alcoholism rehabilitation and can provide the role model that is convincing to alcoholic persons. Nurses, social workers, physicians, and psychologists are relative newcomers to these settings. Their special professional skills and health orientations add greatly to the therapeutic programs. The nurse, in particular, has a unique opportunity to use her skills. Depending on her competencies, she may be the person responsible for the assessment of the client's health status and for providing appropriate intervention or making judgments as to necessary referrals. Furthermore, her participation in the treatment program may include individual and group counseling and providing alcohol-related education.

Alcoholism treatment facilities in the past have focused primarily on the arrest of alcoholism, to the exclusion of coexisting health problems. Although some physiologic disturbances such as fluid and electrolyte imbalances, tremors, nausea, and vomiting become resolved with an increasing period of abstinence, others such as alcohol-related heart disease, pancreatitis, or hepatic disease do not and may require medical and nursing intervention. The presence of nurses with relevant educational preparation within alcoholism treatment facilities helps to bridge this gap. These nurses perform a vital function and are likely to find this work interesting and satisfying.

Alcoholism outpatient clinics

Alcoholism clinics provide treatment to alcoholic persons on an outpatient basis. Such clinics may be free-standing facilities or part of community mental health centers. Additionally, physicians, nurses, social workers, and psychologists in private practice may offer treatment for alcoholism on an outpatient basis.

Outpatient services typically are not operating on a full-time basis; rather, they are limited to work-week hours. Thus in the event of a weekend crisis the client may have to seek help elsewhere.

An outpatient program, by its very nature, requires the alcoholic person to be well enough to reach the facility and to live somewhere else. Thus the clientele seen in outpatient clinics differs from that of inpatient facilities in the degree of physical wellness and socioeconomic status.

Commonly used treatment modalities include individual and group counseling, didactic lectures, and introduction to Alcoholics Anonymous. Many clinics provide family counseling, and often they conduct specialty sessions for women, adolescents, and the elderly.

The treatment staff consist of health professionals (nurses, physicians, social workers, clinical psychologists) and alcoholism counselors. In an outpatient treatment program there is less control over ongoing drinking behavior and less opportunity to interrupt drinking than in inpatient facilities. Thus the alcoholic person who needs, at least temporarily, the external control of being cut off from alcohol will not find it in outpatient therapy. This limits the potential effectiveness of outpatient treatment clinics and may be the reason why dropout rates from these services are high. There is a tendency for the less educated, less motivated, and more socially disrupted persons to drop out before therapeutic relationships have been established.[25] The strength of an alcoholism outpatient clinic lies in its availability to people in the important work it performs with families and specialty groups of alcoholic persons.

Elements affecting behavioral change

From the foregoing it becomes clear that therapeutic approaches used in the management of alcoholic persons are nonspecific. Whereas all approaches have a degree of usefulness with some clients, none is universally effective. Recovery from alcoholism, as has been stated previously, generally requires the alcoholic person to make changes in most all behaviors. Having used alcohol to cope with life situations, the alcoholic now has to learn new and different ways to deal with them. Because available treatment modalities bring about desired changes for some alcoholic persons, it is well to examine elements that are known to affect behavior in general and explore their potential usefulness in understanding behavior of alcoholic persons. Some such elements known to influence human behavior in general and alcoholic persons in particular include reactions to phases of illness, the experience of hope, the nature of the person's self-concept, and the quality of the therapeutic relationship. These elements are examined next for their applicability to alcoholic persons in the process of recovery.

Phases of illness

It has been known for some time that adaptations to conditions requiring changes in behavior occur with time and are governed by specific behavioral reactions. A person experiencing physical disability, for instance, can be expected to encounter phases similar to those described as taking place after a crisis.[11] When normal coping mechanisms are inadequate to deal with the disability, sequential phases of shock, defensive retreat, acknowledgment, and adaptation follow. During the initial period of adaptation, the person tends to feel emotionally numb and unable to formulate plans of action. Gradually, he tries to overcome the overwhelming feeling of shock by shutting out the threat imposed on him. He tries to cling to life as it always has been, denying the existence of the condition and avoiding reality. When he recognizes that life does not return to its former state and that people do not support his unrealistic beliefs, he begins to acknowledge that reality is different, that a change has occurred, and that he cannot fight this change. During the last phase, that of adaptation, the individual develops a renewed sense of worth and begins to explore new resources.[11]

The alcoholic person has been observed to experience these phases of adaptation.[18] In this recurring condition, however, adaptations rarely occur in continuous, sequential patterns. Rather, there is a fluctuation of movement in and out of phases of adaptation. Periods of sobriety, during which acknowledgment of illness and movement toward new ways of life occur, may be followed by relapse and reexperience of shock and denial. Generally, as periods of sobriety lengthen, phases of shock and denial become briefer and acknowledgment and adaptation tend to prevail.

Identification of the illness stage is important and necessary to make effective nursing intervention. Such identification provides a basis for setting realistic goals and for understanding the sometimes puzzling behavior of some patients. During periods of shock and disbelief, support and factual information are most useful to the client. When the person is in the phase of denial, techniques that penetrate this behavior defense are useful. During phases of acceptance and adaptation, the client is most likely to accept guidance that will help him to achieve recovery and rehabilitation.

Hope

The sense of hope to be able to reach new goals is a strong motivating force toward change. It is known that the greater the expectation to attain new goals the more likely the individual will be to act.[32] Conversely, when the expectation to reach a goal is low or absent, people tend to "give up" and may even die. Such conditions were observed in concentration camps[3] and in experimentation on humans and animals.[27] The alcoholic person frequently lacks hope of being able to live without alcohol. Repeated futile attempts to give up alcohol may have resulted in a state of hopelessness. The person believes that friends, relatives, and health professionals have reinforced his feelings in their communications and behavior toward him. They usually indicated disbelief of his ability to effect changes from his alcoholic state.

The nurse can promote feelings of hope in her relationship with the alcoholic person. The nurse's own confidence in an alcoholic person's ability to move toward rehabilitation is important in transmitting expectations of his being able to reach such goals. Furthermore, hope becomes reinforced when the person begins to experience satisfaction from the ability to document day-by-day progress in health, interpersonal relationships, and abstaining from alcohol. Such experiences result from setting short-term, reasonable goals mutually defined and periodically evaluated by client and nurse.

Concept of self

As hopefulness begins to replace feelings of dejection, and as accomplishments toward recovery accumulate, the person's views of himself improve. Self-concept, or the way an individual sees himself in relation to the world around him, is an important determinant of behavior. The alcoholic person has been described as having a low self-concept.[36] Experiences of failure in nearly all ways of living, reinforced by rejection from others important to him, have convinced him of his low value as an individual. Such conceptions hinder actions toward positive changes and tend to perpetuate living styles abusive to personal health on the premise that an individual of low value does not deserve any better.

The informed nurse has the opportunity to influence changes in a client's self-conception. On the basis of the knowledge that alcoholic drinking is not a chosen way of behavior but rather that external and internal circumstances contribute to its development, the nurse can institute deliberate actions aimed at reversing the client's belief about himself. The message conveyed in the relationships with the client is important. As the nurse transmits respect, courtesy, and consideration, the person begins to adopt such views for himself. The nurse further contributes to the enhancement of the self-image by planning achievable goals with the client and by creating an awareness of achievements in overtly calling attention to his accomplishments. As the concept of self improves, planning for changes that promote the person's state of living are more likely to result. Theorists believe that perceptions of self are predictive of human behavior.[39] Hence the person who likes himself can be expected to behave in ways that exhibit self-satisfaction. The nurse can use the knowledge of a client's belief about himself as one basis for planning care and anticipating change.

Helping relationship

As alluded to before, perhaps the most important component in the facilitation of change is the quality of the relationship between nurse and client. A relationship that fosters trust and acceptance and the ability to grow and change is a truly helping relationship. It permits the client to explore freely the problems that have contributed to his alcoholic drinking and the issues that lie ahead in achieving sobriety, health, and general well-being.

The helping relationship is one which demonstrates a sense of caring to the client and a concern for the improvement of his health in an atmosphere of unreserved acceptance.

Of greatest importance to the relationship is the feeling tone that prevails. The alcoholic person, who has experienced long-time rejection and who generally has a low concept of himself, is highly sensitive to the nurse's reactions toward him. He is alert to even subtle nuances of speech and behavior that indicate disdain, and he will withdraw from the nurse when he senses rejection. To protect himself further from perceived rejections, he uses defense mechanisms such as denial. Communication of significant issues under such conditions is not possible.

In contrast, the nurse who accepts the alcoholic client as she does any other client, and who understands that alcoholism is treatable, creates an atmosphere in which the alcoholic person feels supported. He can relax his defenses and is free to examine options that may lead to rehabilitation.

The helping relationship is a caring relationship. It is one in which the growth of the alcoholic client, from one of dependence on alcohol to one of more normal functioning becomes an important concern. It involves heightened awareness and increased responsiveness to the needs of the client. It means that the nurse attempts to understand the client and his world as he views it and as he sees himself; it means seeing what life is like for the alcoholic person, what he is striving to be, and what he requires to grow.[23]

Caring is in evidence when the nurse takes time to talk with the client, when she listens to him, and when she acts on his behalf. It is present when she responds to his needs at times when he most experiences them rather than at scheduled hours. The nurse exhibits caring also when she views difficult behavior of the alcoholic client in the context of the client's coping with alcoholism. All these and other behavior tell the alcoholic person that the nurse indeed cares, and perhaps so do others close to him.

The helping relationship is health oriented. This means that the improvement of the client's state of well-being is of central concern. The alcoholic client must learn to understand and accept that he has alcoholism and that it is a chronic progressive condition; he must learn to understand what it is he must and can do to halt its progression. Armed with knowledge about alcoholism and with an understanding of the client, the nurse confronts the alcoholic person with factual information in a manner that he can understand and accept and use. A health-oriented relationship requires the nurse to oppose the client's views, beliefs, and actions, when these are contrary to known tenets of health, even at the risk of an affront. In the presence of a genuine relationship, it is often possible for the client to accept a painful truth without feeling the need to retaliate. The helping relationship is one which makes it possible for the alcoholic person to change and grow. It has been described as one which will allow the client to discover within himself the capacity to use that relationship for growth, change, and personal development.[28]

REFERENCES

1. Alcoholics Anonymous, ed. 2, New York, 1955, Alcoholics Anonymous World Services, Inc.
2. Benson, H.: Decreased alcohol intake associated with the practice of meditation: a retrospective investigation. In Seixas, F. A., et al., editors: Annals of the New York Academy of Sciences **233**:174, 1974.

3. Bettelheim, B.: The informed heart, Glencoe, Ill., 1960, Free Press.
4. Blane, H. T.: Psychotherapeutic approach. In Kissin, B., and Begleiter, H., editors: The biology of alcoholism, Vol. 5, Treatment and rehabilitation of the chronic alcoholic, New York, 1977, Plenum Press, Inc.
5. Brothers, J.: Joan Kennedy's road back from alcoholism, Good Housekeeping, p. 106, April, 1979.
6. Cain, A.: The role of the therapist in family systems therapy, The Family 3:65, 1976.
7. Cole, J., and Ryback, R.: Pharmacological Therapy. In Tarter, R., and Sugarman, A. A.: Alcoholism, Reading, Mass., 1976, Addison-Wesley Publishing Co., Inc.
8. Corrigan, E. M.: Linking the problem drinker with treatment, Social Work 17:54, 1972.
9. Curlee-Salisbury, J.: Perspectives on Alcoholics Anonymous. In Estes, N. J., and Heinemann, M. E., editors: Alcoholism, development, consequences, and interventions, St. Louis, 1977, The C. V. Mosby Co.
10. Edwards, G., et al.: Alcoholism a controlled trial of "treatment" and "advice," Journal of Studies on Alcohol 38:1004, 1977.
11. Fink, S. L.: Crisis and motivation: a theoretical model, Archives of Physical Medicine and Rehabilitation, 48:592, 1967.
12. Fox, V.: Recognizing multiple simultaneous drug withdrawal syndromes. Presented to NCA/AMSA Medical-Scientific Conference, Washington, D.C., May 6-8, 1976.
13. Gary, V., and Guthrie, D.: The effect of jogging on physical fitness and self-concept in hospitalized alcoholics, Quarterly Journal of Studies on Alcohol 33:1073, 1972.
14. Green, E., Green, A. M., and Walters, E. D.: Biofeedback training for anxiety tension reduction, Annals of the New York Academy of Sciences 233:157, 1974.
15. Kissin, B.: Patient characteristics and treatment specificity in alcoholism. In Mello, N. K., and Mendelson, J. H., editors: Recent advances in studies of alcoholism, Rockville, Md., 1971, Publication no. (HSM) 71-9045, U.S. Government Printing Office.
16. Kissin, B.: Theory and practice in the treatment of alcoholism. In Kissin, B., and Begleiter, H., editors: The biology of alcoholism, Vol. 5, Treatment and rehabilitation of the chronic alcoholic, New York, 1977, Plenum Press, Inc.
17. Kline, N. S., et al.: Evaluation of lithium therapy in chronic and periodic alcoholism, American Journal of Medical Sciences 268:15, 1974.
18. Lambert, D.: Difficulties in accepting the diagnosis of alcoholism. In Selected Papers, 22nd Annual Meeting, Sept. 12-17, 1971, Hartford, Conn., Alcohol and Drug Problems Association of North America.
19. Lemere, F., and Voegtlin, W. L.: An evaluation of the aversion treatment of alcoholism, Quarterly Journal of Studies on Alcohol 4:199, 1950.
20. Marlatt, A. G., and Gordon, J. R.: Determinants of relapse: implications for the maintenance of behavior change. In Davidson, P., editor: Behavioral medicine: changing health life style, New York, 1979, Brunner/Mazel, Inc.
21. Marlatt, A., and Nathan, P.: Behavioral approaches to alcoholism, New Brunswick, N.J., 1978, Rutgers Center of Alcohol Studies.
22. Materi, M.: Assertiveness training: a catalyst for behavioral change, Alcohol Health and Research World, 1:23, Summer, 1977.
23. Mayeroff, M.: On caring, New York, 1971, Perennial Library, Harper & Row Publishers.
24. O'Briant, R., Peterson, N. W., and Heacock, D.: How safe is social setting detoxification? Alcohol Health and Research World 1:22, 1976/1977.
25. Pattison, M.: Rehabilitation of the chronic alcoholic. In Kissin, B., and Begleiter, H., editors: The biology of alcoholism, Vol. 3, Clinical pathology, New York, 1974, Plenum Press, Inc.

26. Plaut, T. F. A.: Alcohol problems: a report to the nation, New York, 1967, Oxford University Press.
27. Richter, C. P.: On the phenomenon of sudden death in animals and man, Psychosomatic medicine **19**:191, 1957.
28. Rogers, C.: On becoming a person, Boston, 1961, Houghton Mifflin Co.
29. Scott, E. M.: Struggles in an alcoholic family, Springfield, Ill., 1970, Charles C Thomas, Publisher.
30. Solberg, R. J.: The dry-drunk syndrome, Center City, Minn., Hazelden Foundation.
31. Smith-DiJulio, K., Heinemann, M. E., and Ogden, L.: Diagnosis and care of the alcoholic patient during acute episodes. In Estes, N. J., and Heinemann, M. E., editors: Alcoholism, development, consequences, and interventions, St. Louis, 1977, The C. V. Mosby Co.
32. Stotland, E.: The psychology of hope, San Francisco, 1969, Jossey-Bass, Inc., Publishers.
33. Thompson, W. L., et al.: Diazepam and paraldehyde for treatment of severe delirium tremens: a controlled trial, Annals of Internal Medicine **82**:175, 1975.
34. United States Department of Health, Education, and Welfare: First special report to U.S. Congress on alcohol and health, DHEW Publication no. (HSM) 72-9099, Washington, D.C., 1971, U.S. Government Printing Office.
35. United States Department of Health, Education and Welfare: Third special report to U.S. Congress on alcohol and health, DHEW Publication no. (ADM) 78-569, Washington, D.C., 1978, U.S. Government Printing Office.
36. Vanderpool, J. A.: Alcoholism and the self concept, Quarterly Journal of Studies on Alcohol **30**:59, 1969.
37. Weinberg, J.: Counseling the person with alcohol problems: In Estes, N. J., and Heinemann, M. E., editors: Alcoholism, development, consequences, and interventions, St. Louis, 1977, The C. V. Mosby Co.
38. Whyte, C. R., and O'Brien, P. M. J.: Disulfiram implant: a controlled trial, British Journal of Psychiatry **124**:42, 1974.
39. Wylie, R.: The self concept, Lincoln, Nebr., 1961, University of Nebraska Press.
40. Zimberg, S., Wallace, J., and Blume, S.: Practical approaches to alcoholism psychotherapy, New York, 1978, Plenum Press, Inc.

CHAPTER 11

Family members of the alcoholic person

Alcoholism has been called the "family illness" because of its potentially injurious impact on all members of the family unit. The spouse of the alcoholic person becomes deeply troubled as the pervasive and painful effects of alcoholism gradually impinge on the marital relationship. As the alcoholic person's excessive drinking increases, the spouse experiences many conflicting feelings and becomes involved in efforts to manage the growing chaos within the family. These efforts, ranging from ignoring the drinking to intensive efforts to control it, although well intended, often lead to a perpetuation or acceleration of the excessive drinking.

Children are especially vulnerable to the adverse effects of parental alcoholism. They rarely possess the skill for understanding or handling the discord within their homes and frequently become victims of emotional neglect and family conflict.

Some family members directly seek professional help for alcohol-related problems. More likely the concerns of family members surface when, as a part of routine health appraisal, nurses are alert and responsive to evidence that alcohol-related problems are troublesome to their clients. Whether such persons are identified directly or indirectly, nurses need to understand the dynamics of families with alcoholism, to have skill in appraising spouses and children from homes with alcoholism, and to know where to refer them for help. To assist the nurse in achieving these goals, this chapter presents two contrasting models for understanding the dynamics of alcoholism in families and appraisal approaches for spouses and children. Examples of community resources appropriate to the needs of families with an alcoholic member are also given.

MODELS FOR UNDERSTANDING ALCOHOLISM IN THE FAMILY

Families are not affected equally by alcoholism. In some, alcoholism becomes the central feature around which family life ensues, and in others it is only of little importance to total family interaction. In either case, families who remain intact evolve ways of maintaining themselves in the presence of an alcoholic member. Two frameworks that elaborate on the dynamics of family interaction with an alcoholic member and that provide alternate means for organizing and analyzing relevant appraisal data are stress and systems theories.

Stress theory

The sociologic perspective is the conceptual foundation on which stress theory is based. The sociologic approach to the alcoholic marriage emphasizes the structure, process, and functions of the family unit. It concentrates on institutionalized regulations that control families and ways in which marriage partners behave in their cultural roles. The sociologic perspective is concerned with how the marital pair reacts under certain social conditions and transition states and to environmental stress.[35]

The landmark papers on the sociologic stress theory and the family with alcoholism were published several decades ago.[21-24] Even so, aspects of this literature are still widely cited in alcoholism counseling literature, regularly used in Al-Anon discussion groups, and republished in current alcoholism texts. Some of these formulations are presented here because they provide a valid way of understanding the adjustment of the family to an alcoholic member.

In the framework of stress theory, alcoholism is considered to be a personal condition belonging to the excessively drinking person rather than being a property of the marriage or family. It is recognized, however, that the alcoholism has profound implications for the family.[33] It is assumed that family relationships deteriorate as a consequence of the strain of living with an alcoholic member and that improvement in family interaction occurs when the drinker stops or modifies his behavior. Alcoholism is seen as a source of stress or crisis to which family members react by experiencing critical stages of adjustment or by developing specific coping behavior.[21,26,34] A crisis can be defined as a condition of acute anxiety occurring when someone's usual ways of coping are no longer adequate and new solutions are needed.[15]

The family behavior that evolves when the alcoholic member is a husband and father is presented as a special case of family crisis.[24] Progressive events occur as follows. When people live together over a period of time, patterns of relating and behaving as a unit evolve. Families divide functions and have interlocking roles. For the family to function smoothly, members must enact their roles in a predictable manner and according to the family expectations. When the family as a unit is functioning smoothly, individual members as a rule function well. Members are aware of where they fit, what they are expected to do, and what can be expected from others. When these expectations are not met, repercussions are felt by every family member, and the family as a whole ceases to function smoothly. A crisis is under way.

Regardless of the precipitating factors, family crises follow a pattern.[24] First, there is denial that a problem exists. Second, when denial is no longer effective, there is a downward slump in organization, roles are played with less enthusiasm, and tensions and strained relationships increase. Third, as the family finds some successful technique of adjustment, it stabilizes at a new level. Fourth, as the crisis continues, roles of family members change, there is an alteration in the perception of self and others, and considerable mental conflict is experienced by all involved.

In a family, when one of the adults becomes an alcoholic, a cumulative crisis pattern develops in response to the alcoholism, but the crisis is complicated by recurrent subsidiary crises such as unemployment, impoverishment, and desertion. In addition to this complicated interrelationship of crises, the nonalcoholic spouse often feels that there is no one to turn to for help. As a result, the crisis is handled by techniques of trial and error.

Research with nonalcoholic spouses of male alcoholics has suggested that families experience seven stages of adjustment to the crises or stress of alcoholism.[21] The first stage of adjustment involves *attempts to deny the problem*. As sporadic incidents of excessive drinking occur, strain is placed on husband-wife interactions, but the couple attempts to minimize the episodes by denying their seriousness or that they occurred at all. In an attempt to minimize drinking, problems in marital adjustment not related to alcohol are avoided.

The second stage involves *attempts to eliminate the problem*. In this stage, as incidents of excessive drinking multiply, the family begins to engage in social isolation to decrease the visibility of the drinker to others. The isolation magnifies the importance of the family interactions and events, and much of what is discussed in the home is alcohol centered. Tensions rise, and the husband-wife relationship deteriorates. The wife may feel sorry for herself and lose self-confidence as her efforts to control her husband's drinking repeatedly fail. The children begin to show evidence of emotional disturbance as family interaction is disrupted anew with each episode of drinking.

In the third stage, *disorganization*, chaos is at its peak. It is manifested by inept communication, role distortion, and sexual dysfunction. Family members give up attempts to control the drinking and begin behaving in a manner designed to relieve immediate tensions rather than attempting achievement of long-term goals. The drinker's roles as husband and father are no longer supported, and disturbances on the part of the children multiply. The wife wonders about her sanity and worries about her ability to make decisions and to change the situation.

The fourth stage, *attempts to reorganize in spite of the problem*, involves efforts by the wife to take over control of the family. She tries to ignore her husband as much as possible or treats him like a recalcitrant child. He is seen as more dependent than dependable. The wife may feel pity for her husband and strongly protective of him during this phase rather than resentful and hostile as in earlier phases. As the wife succeeds in bringing some semblance of order to family life, her self-confidence begins to be rebuilt.

The fifth stage, *efforts to escape the problem,* involves separation of the wife and children from the drinker. Some wives have great difficulty resolving the problems and conflicts surrounding separation and/or divorce, so this stage may be delayed or never achieved.

Reorganization of part of the family is described in the sixth stage, when the wife and children reorganize as a family without the husband and father.

The seventh and final stage, *recovery and reorganization of the whole family,* occurs if the husband achieves sobriety. The family decides to reunite to include the sober husband and father. Many families experience problems in adjusting to his presence. Some alcoholic persons in the throes of learning to live without alcohol may be even more difficult to live with than when they were drinking.

Five major problem areas encountered by a group of wives during the early stages of their husband's sobriety have been described.[14] The first area, *reinstatement of the husband into family roles,* entails the reestablishment of family relationships based on mutual trust and resumption by the husband of responsibilities connected with being a spouse and father. A second area involves *difficulties surrounding communication.* Disruptive patterns of communicating, inculcated during the drinking phase, are difficult to change and replace with satisfactory, congruent patterns. The third major problem area, *affective responses of the wife,* includes her tendency to experience fears, diminished self-worth, bouts of depression, and lingering resentments. The fourth area consists of *traits and behaviors of the husband found to be particularly disruptive to the wife,* including his tendency to be evasive, egocentric, moody, irresponsive, and overly sensitive. It also includes the syndrome of "dry drunk," a term describing the state of the alcoholic person who is extremely uncomfortable when not drinking. *Handling situations involving alcohol or alcohol-related problems* comprises the final problem area. It includes concerns about the maintenance of sobriety in a drinking society, such as responding to blandishments and comments about the refusal to drink.

These problem areas indicate that sobriety does not in itself bring instant happiness to the family who has lived for years with an alcoholic member. Rather, old problems linger and new ones emerge as the family attempts to reunite.

As stated earlier, a second way of studying families experiencing the stress of alcoholism involves identifying the coping behavior instituted by nonalcoholic members. Five reasonably distinct and persistent styles of coping behavior utilized by wives of alcoholic husbands include withdrawal within marriage, protection, attack, safeguarding family interests, and acting out.[34] Various specific behaviors on the wife's part are associated with each coping style. *Withdrawal within marriage*, the most frequently used style of coping, includes quarrels about drinking, evading the husband, sexual withdrawal, and avoidance of the wife's own feelings. *Protection* involves pouring out the liquor, insisting that the husband eat, and interceding with the employer on the husband's behalf. The third style, *attack*, includes discussion about divorce and locking the husband out of the house. *Safeguarding family interests* involves paying debts, hiding the husband's money, and keeping the children out of his way. In the final coping style, *acting out*, the wife gets drunk in an attempt to control her husband's drinking, makes him jealous, and threatens suicide.

The wife's coping styles change over time, depending on the stage of the husband's drinking and the behavior the husband is manifesting.[26] All wives use more than one style at one time or another, and all the styles reach a peak during the husband's periods of heaviest drinking.

Whether through adaptive stages or by developing different coping styles, the family with an alcoholic member attempts to achieve adjustment and stabilization. These efforts are seen by stress theory proponents as a reaction to the strain of alcoholism as it invades the family unit and interferes with its smooth functioning.

Systems theory

A second and relatively new model for understanding alcoholism in the family is systems theory. General systems theory integrates knowledge from a number of sciences, including biology, cybernetics, economics, communications, psychology, and operations research. Although there is some overlap between stress and systems theory, the stress model emphasizes alcoholism as a personal condition belonging to the excessive drinker rather than to the family. Systems theory, on the other hand, emphasizes interactional issues and changing relationships and interrelationships within the family, spanning several generations such as grandparents, parents, and children.

The family as a system is dynamic, with constant interactional exchange occurring among its members. Each member is interdependent on the others. If one member is not functioning well, all family members will be affected. In the family with alcoholism the excessive drinker is viewed as the signaler of some distress in the system. He is not blamed for the disruption, nor are others in the family blamed for the alcoholic person's suffering. In fact, blaming has no useful place in systems theory. All important people within the family are seen as contributing to the way in which family members relate to each other and in the way that symptoms finally erupt.[7] Thus, in systems theory, to comprehend individual behavior, it is necessary to understand the family in which the person lives, the relationships within the family, and the importance of each individual's behavior in maintaining the family system. The family is seen as the troubled unit rather than an individual, and solutions to difficulties must be sought at the system or family level, not at the subsystem or individual level.

Observable facts of relationships are the focus of systems theory. Studying what, how, when, and where interactions take place always has precedence over analyzing why an interaction or family event occurred. Therefore, in a family with an alcoholic member, the systems theorist would explore what is happening in family interactions, how the interactions come about, when the behaviors of individual members occur in an attempt to understand how alcoholism developed within the family, and how alcoholism is being maintained by the family.

The notion that the whole is more than the sum of its parts is a central feature of systems theory. In other words the totality of a family as an operating system is greater than the sum of the persons within the family. It is a larger whole when viewed together and is composed of internal dyads, triads, and complex groupings. The family members are often in intense relationships that constantly interact and change. The shifting and changing are attempts by the parts of the system to maintain a state of balance or homeostasis. Homeostasis is the inclination of a system to maintain a dynamic equilibrium around some central tendency and to undertake operations designed to restore that equilibrium when it is threatened in some way.[4] Dynamic equilibrium reflects an adjustment that is successful and satisfactory in some way or to some degree to family members. The level of adjustment may not appear to be the best to outsiders, but once a family has achieved an internal balance it resists modification. There is a constant effort to maintain the status quo by reacting against any change.

All persons within a family system are engaged in stability maintenance or homeostasis. When a change occurs within one family member, there must be a compensatory change in the other members. This action-reaction mechanism is known as feedback.[28]

Feedback may be negative or positive. *Negative feedback* tends to provide a restraining force to a system and moves it toward stability. *Positive feedback* tends to promote further activity and moves a system toward instability.[11] It can act like a thermostat that has become stuck and is constantly calling for more heat. Unless limited, positive feedback can create sufficient alterations to destroy the system. Negative feedback, on the other hand, can maintain homeostasis and correct errors and deviations.[18]

When a system is functioning smoothly, no particular difficulties are encountered with positive feedback. If, on the other hand, there is a signal of system disruption, as when a family member develops alcoholism, positive feedback may create further instability as depicted in the following example. A wife in the family developed alcoholism and began incurring numerous debts. The husband, to compensate for the indebtedness, cancelled the children's music lessons to pay for the groceries and took a second job to pay other bills formerly covered by a single paycheck. These actions unwittingly enabled the wife to have more money available for alcohol and alcohol-related activities, thus perpetuating her further involvement in alcoholism. Eventually, positive feedback in this situation resulted in a runaway situation as the wife spent more and more money to maintain her excessive use of alcohol. In response, both the husband and children initiated additional ways of acquiring more money themselves and stretching the available dollars further in an effort to regain financial homeostasis.

Negative feedback, on the other hand, calls for a change in the direction of the system. It promotes the development of equilibrium and stability when system disruption has occurred by dislodging a system from an equilibrium that is functionally stale and nonproductive for its members.[3] In the previous example, if the husband refused to take a second job or to compensate in any way for the indebtedness, the wife would more likely face the consequences of her drinking and choose whether to continue it or not. If the wife were to receive multiple negative feedback from a variety of systems, such as friends, extended family, or mortgage company and other creditors, the likelihood that she will discontinue drinking is increased. When the negative feedback leads to cessation of drinking, the family is in a better position to reestablish itself into a functioning, productive system again. Systems, such as the family, are constantly faced with new challenges and, to remain in balance, are in a constant state of flux.[28]

The family system is made up not only of interrelated parts but is itself an interrelated part of larger systems. Some examples of larger systems to which families are interrelated include school, work, neighborhood, and community systems. These larger systems provide feedback to the family, thereby influencing its functioning. The extent to which the family can exchange feedback within itself and with its external systems depends on at least two aspects: the family's ability to perform its basic functions and the extent to which the family system is open or closed.

Family systems have several basic functions. These include *maintaining balanced relationships* among members of the family and *performing the duties* for which the family was devised, such as nurturing the young, meeting the physical and emotional needs of its members, transmitting the culture, and relating to the environment. If most of the energy of the family is used in maintaining balanced relationships, there will be little energy left for growth of the family as a whole or of its individual members or for accommodating feedback from systems outside itself. Systems do not create new energy; they only move the available energy around. If too much energy is used in attaining one function, there will be a deficit when energy is needed elsewhere.

The other aspect of the family's ability to exchange feedback internally and externally has to do with the extent to which the family system is open or closed. There is no completely open or closed system when applied to families; rather, they differ in degrees of openness. It is well to keep this factor in mind when studying theory about open and closed family systems.

Closed family systems are characterized by low feelings of self-worth; unclear, growth-impeding communication patterns; and covert, rigid rules for behavior leading to accidental or destructive outcomes. In a family that operates as a closed system, the self-worth of the members becomes increasingly uncertain.[36] The family with an alcoholic member provides an example of a closed system. When the mother in a family has alcoholism, much of the energy of the family members may be devoted to trying to compel her to perform her expected roles. Repeated arguments and threats directed at the mother, especially on the part of her husband, may leave little time or energy for nurturing activities or for dealing with input from outside systems such as responding to a teacher's observation that one of the children is having learning problems.

On the other hand, *open family systems* are more able to fulfill their basic functions. In them the self-worth of the members is high and communication is direct, clear, and growth producing. The rules for behavior are overt and change when the need arises. The outcome for family members is related to reality and is appropriate and constructive. The self-worth of those within an open system becomes increasingly more reliable and confident.[36]

The perspective of systems theory, systematically applied to alcoholic marriages, is relatively new and still evolving. The findings of several such studies are presented to illustrate application of systems theory to the marriage and/or family with alcoholism.

In studying the alcoholic person and his helpers, such as family members and employers, it was found that many repetitive interactions occur between a pathologic drinker and others which provide positive reinforcement of drinking.[38] Predominant among these interactions were those concerned with denial of the alcoholic problem and punishment and/or forgiveness of the drinker following intoxication. With time these interactions become circular, entrenched, and self-perpetuating, thus adding continuous invigoration to the drinking behavior and causing difficulty in changing the status quo. This action-reaction (i.e., excessive drinking on the part of the alcoholic person followed by punishment by nonalcoholic family members) is typical of positive feedback that tends to maintain a closed family system. Much of the energy of the family is used to fulfill the task of attempting to maintain balanced relationships between members of the family, and little, if any, is left for growth-producing functions.

In another study responsibility-avoiding behavior has been identified as the key behavior used by the alcoholic person, drunk or sober, as a means of indirectly controlling others.[16] The alcoholic person accomplishes this control by being ambiguous, confusing, and inconsistent and by shifting responsibility for his actions to others. When the spouse of the alcoholic accepts this irresponsibility, and sometimes even promotes it, the status quo of the alcoholic person's having control over the relationship will be maintained. If there is an escalation of conflict over who has control and the alcoholic person thinks he is losing, he restabilizes the system through further drinking. The excessive drinking is seen as a rigid, circular behavior used by the alcoholic person to maintain control of the family.

A final example of the application of systems theory to families with alcoholism again emphasizes how family interaction affects excessive drinking.[7] Family members who are most dependent on the drinking person are more overtly anxious than the one who drinks. The way in which family members relate to each other proceeds in a circular pattern as follows. The more the family is threatened by the drinking the more anxious they become. As anxiety increases, so does their tendency to criticize the drinker, which in turn escalates emotional isolation. As a result the alcoholic member drinks more, which feeds into the spiraling problem of increased anxiety, criticism, and emotional distance within the family. The problem worsens, and both sides become more rigidly self-righteous. Anything that will interrupt the increasing anxiety will be helpful. Any one significant family member who can control his or her own anxiety can make a step toward de-escalation.

In summary, systems theory emphasizes that family units need to function smoothly. When something interferes with that functioning, the family struggles to reestablish homeostasis. This striving for homeostasis can lead to behaviors that resist change over long periods of time. In the context of the alcoholic person and his family, excessive drinking behavior, once established, becomes part of the status quo. The alcoholism is often unwittingly perpetuated by the behavior of family members. At the same time, systems theory emphasizes that it is possible for growth-producing change to occur within the family unit when members learn to make affirmative alterations in their responses.

APPRAISAL OF THE SPOUSE

As the nurse appraises nonalcoholic family members such as the spouse in various health care settings, she needs an understanding of the processes just described, which occur with some regularity in homes with an alcoholic member. With this understanding the nurse will identify clues in the spouse's behavior that indicate alcohol-related problems, administer screening tools when indicated, and if diagnosis is made, promote a dialogue surrounding the concerns of the person and make appropriate referrals.

Clues to alcohol-related problems

Some spouses who seek health care for themselves for various reasons will state openly during the appraisal process that they have an alcoholic mate. More often such information will be revealed only after keen observation and sensitive inquiry by the nurse.

Spouses who do not directly acknowledge that they have an alcoholic mate may do so indirectly by talking about matters related to associated family difficulties. These include economic impairments, sexual maladjustments, separation and divorce, quarreling, violence, complaints about feeling isolated and lonely, and expressions of resentment about having to carry the bulk of responsibility for child rearing and discipline. In addition, to compensate for feeling overwhelmed with alcohol-related problems, parental responsibilities are shifted to older childen in the family or to relatives, friends, and neighbors outside the home. Some spouses express vague fears of insanity, mention thoughts of suicide for undisclosed reasons, or manifest great difficulty in decision making.

One woman seeking care because of excessive vaginal bleeding between menstrual periods became anxious when further diagnostic tests were suggested. She repeatedly sought verbal reassurance that her problem was not malignant. Finally, with obvious embarrassment, she confided that because of financial indebtedness within her family she could not afford any further testing. The nurse, knowing that the client was married and unemployed outside the home, asked about the nature of her husband's work. She was told that he held a well-paying position with a reputable firm. Noting the discrepancy between the family income and indebtedness, coupled with the woman's embarrassment and anxiety in discussing her situation, the nurse asked the client what was contributing to her financial and emotional difficulties. The woman paused and finally breathed a deep sigh of relief and said, "Alcohol!" She subsequently described her husband's long-term involvement with drinking and the myriad problems his excessive alcohol use had produced within the family. After conferring further with other health team members about finances, she left with appointments for further gynecologic examination and for in-depth assessment of the alcoholism in her family.

Whenever the nurse becomes suspicious about the client's behavior, as in the situation just described, because matters seem incongruous, it is well to pursue further questioning. If the nurse's knowledge and observations lead her to suspect that alcohol is involved in the person's dilemma, it is advisable to ask directly. A statement like, "Is alcohol playing any part in the difficulties you are experiencing?" is usually appropriate.

Questionnaires for appraisal

Some spouses with an alcoholic mate will benefit from filling out a paper and pencil test as an initial means of communicating about their experiences. A written tool is neutral and objectively indicates whether a problem actually exists. Such a measure is a highly acceptable way of obtaining information and can provide considerable relief from the highly emotional, subjective exchanges that most likely have transpired many times between family members surrounding the subject of alcoholism.

One such tool is entitled "The Family 20-Question Questionnaire,"[20] shown here, and includes questions that are answered "Yes" or "No."

THE FAMILY 20-QUESTION QUESTIONNAIRE*

Ask yourself these questions about your husband's or your wife's drinking

1.	Do you worry about your spouse's drinking?	Yes ☐	No ☐
2.	Have you ever been embarrassed by your spouse's drinking?	Yes ☐	No ☐
3.	Are holidays more of a nightmare than a celebration because of your spouse's drinking behavior?	Yes ☐	No ☐
4.	Are most of your spouse's friends heavy drinkers?	Yes ☐	No ☐
5.	Does your spouse often promise to quit drinking without success?	Yes ☐	No ☐
6.	Does your spouse's drinking make the atmosphere in the home tense and anxious?	Yes ☐	No ☐
7.	Does your spouse deny a drinking problem because your spouse only drinks beer?	Yes ☐	No ☐
8.	Do you find it necessary to lie to employer, relatives, or friends in order to hide your spouse's drinking?	Yes ☐	No ☐
9.	Has your spouse ever failed to remember what occurred during a drinking period?	Yes ☐	No ☐
10.	Does your spouse avoid conversation pertaining to alcohol or problem drinking?	Yes ☐	No ☐
11.	Does your spouse justify his or her drinking problem?	Yes ☐	No ☐
12.	Does your spouse avoid social situations where alcoholic beverages will not be served?	Yes ☐	No ☐
13.	Do you ever feel guilty about your spouse's drinking?	Yes ☐	No ☐

*Copyright 1976 Donald and Nancy Howard, Box 1362, Columbia, Mo 65201. Reprinted with permission.

14. Has your spouse ever driven a vehicle while under the influence of alcohol?   Yes ☐   No ☐

15. Are your children afraid of your spouse while he or she is drinking?   Yes ☐   No ☐

16. Are you afraid of physical or verbal abuse when your spouse is drinking?   Yes ☐   No ☐

17. Has another person mentioned your spouse's unusual drinking behavior?   Yes ☐   No ☐

18. Do you fear riding with your spouse when he or she is drinking?   Yes ☐   No ☐

19. Does your spouse have periods of remorse after a drinking occasion and apologize for behavior?   Yes ☐   No ☐

20. Do you notice your spouse is getting drunk on fewer drinks?   Yes ☐   No ☐

If you have answered *Yes* to any two of the questions, there is a definite warning that a drinking problem may exist in your family.

If you have answered *Yes* to any four of the questions, the chances are that a drinking problem does exist in your family.

If you have answered *Yes* to five or more, there very definitely is a drinking problem in your family.

The questionnaire focuses on a variety of ways in which alcoholism may be affecting a marriage.

The *feelings of the spouse* regarding the drinker are obtained in the following questions:

1. Do you worry about your husband's drinking?
2. Have you ever been embarrassed by your spouse's drinking?
13. Do you ever feel guilty about your spouse's drinking?
16. Are you afraid of physical or verbal abuse when your spouse is drinking?
18. Do you fear riding with your spouse when he or she is drinking?

The *spouse's beliefs* about the effect of drinking on family events and interactions are covered in questions 3, 6, and 15.

3. Are holidays more of a nightmare than a celebration because of your spouse's drinking behavior?
6. Does your spouse's drinking make the atmosphere in the home tense and anxious?
15. Are your children afraid of your spouse while he or she is drinking?

Inquiries into the *behavior of the drinker* make up the bulk of the questionnaire and are covered in the following questions:

4. Are most of your spouse's friends heavy drinkers?
5. Does your spouse often promise to quit drinking without success?

7. Does your spouse deny a drinking problem because your spouse only drinks beer?
9. Has your spouse ever failed to remember what occurred during a drinking period?
10. Does your spouse avoid conversation pertaining to alcohol or problem drinking?
11. Does your spouse justify his or her drinking problem?
12. Does your spouse avoid social situations where alcoholic beverages will not be served?
14. Has your spouse ever driven a vehicle while under the influence of alcohol?
19. Does your spouse have periods of remorse after a drinking occasion and apologize for behavior?
20. Do you notice your spouse is getting drunk on fewer drinks?

The *behavioral response* of the *spouse* to the mate's drinking is queried in question 8.

8. Do you find it necessary to lie to employer, relatives, or friends in order to hide your spouse's drinking?

The *response of others* outside the family to the drinker's behavior is examined in question 17.

17. Has another person mentioned your spouse's unusual drinking behavior?

A second tool, "22 Questions That Can Help Decide if Someone Close Has a Drinking Problem,"[37] is also designed to help a person decide if someone close has a drinking problem. It contains twenty two yes-no questions, eighteen of which focus on how the *family member feels* about or *responds* to the problem drinker. The remaining four questions ask about the *drinker's behavior* and the *effects on the children* by the drinking. A "yes" answer to any three of the questions indicates that someone else's drinking is exerting a negative influence on the person answering.

22 QUESTIONS THAT CAN HELP DECIDE IF SOMEONE CLOSE HAS A DRINKING PROBLEM*

Answer "yes" or "no":

1. Do most of your thoughts revolve around the problem drinker or problems that arise because of him or her?
2. Do you worry or lose sleep because of a problem drinker?
3. Do you exact promises which are not kept about the amount or how often they are drinking?
4. Do you make threats or decisions and not follow through on them?

---

*Reprinted with permission from Reflect, A Publication of The Dallas Council on Alcoholism, June, 1977. (The 22 questions are a compendium taken from issues of The Utah Alcoholism Foundation Newsletters.)

5. Have you ever lied for or protected them because of their drinking?
6. Do you experience attitude changes toward this problem drinker such as alternating between love and hate?
7. Do you think that everything would be O.K. if only the problem drinker would stop or control the drinking?
8. Do you feel alone—fearful—anxious—angry—or frustrated most of the time? Are you beginning to feel dislike for yourself and to wonder about your sanity?
9. Do you find your moods fluctuating wildly—as a direct result of the problem drinker's moods and actions?
10. Do you feel responsible and guilty about the drinking problem?
11. Are you having any financial difficulties because of drinking and forced to take over more control of family expenditures?
12. Does their drinking keep them away from home a great deal?
13. Is drinking involved in almost all your social activities?
14. Have you withdrawn from outside activities and friends because of embarrassment and shame over the drinking problem?
15. Have you taken over many chores and duties that you would normally expect the problem drinker to assume—or that were formerly his or hers?
16. Do you feel the need to justify your actions and attitudes and, at the same time, feel somewhat smug and self-righteous compared to the drinker?
17. Do you sometimes feel that drinking is more important to them than you are?
18. If there are children in the house, do they often take sides with either the problem drinker or the spouse?
19. Are the children showing signs of emotional stress, such as—withdrawing—having trouble with authority figures—rebelling—acting-out sexually?
20. Have you noticed physical symptoms in yourself, such as—nausea—a "knot" in the stomach—ulcers—shakiness—sweating palms—bitten fingernails?
21. Do you feel utterly defeated—that nothing you can say or do will move the problem drinker? Do you believe that he or she can't get better?
22. Where this applies, is your sexual relationship with a problem drinker affected by feelings of revulsion; do you "use" sex to manipulate—or refuse sex to punish him or her?

Answering *Yes* to any three questions indicates an alcoholism problem in someone else that is exerting negative changes in the person answering.

The two preceding tools, although designed for a similar purpose, provide contrasting data. The first tool emphasizes observations that family members have made about the problem drinker's behavior, whereas the second tool asks family members to examine their feelings about the drinker and how they have behaved in response.

Promoting a dialogue

After the family member, usually a spouse, has completed the questionnaire, the nurse needs to discuss the scoring and the answers provided in some detail with this person. The nature of the questions in each tool will direct the dialogue to a certain degree. As stated previously, the first tool will help the spouse identify more clearly observations made about the drinker, whereas the second tool promotes a discussion of how the spouse feels about and reacts to the drinking behavior.

Most spouses who have been living with an excessive drinker over time will be encumbered with sorrow, regret, and confusion. They often are attempting to fulfill most of the roles in the family—those of provider, parents, decision maker, and homemaker. Many spouses feel resentful about their burdens and have misgivings about how well they are functioning. It is not unusual for them to be susceptible to a great deal of blame placing, fault finding, and accusation when they first have an opportunity to talk with a helping person about their situation.[12]

It is well for the nurse to listen calmly and allow the spouse to experience the cathartic value of speaking freely about an extremely distressing matter. After attentive listening the nurse can assure the spouse that these feelings and responses are similar to those of others living in a comparable situation. The behavior and experiences of the drinker, such as blackouts, denial, and broken promises, can be explained as part of the symptomatology of alcoholism. If the spouse can begin to sense that she is not entirely alone and that the drinker's behavior is often defensive and symptomatic rather than as a result of meanness, lies, or laziness, she may be less judgmental and vengeful. In such a state of mind the spouse is more likely to be responsive to involvement in constructive problem-solving measures.

Some spouses will benefit from clarification of their attitudes and beliefs about alcohol. This can be accomplished by asking the spouse about her life history concerning use or nonuse of alcohol and those close to her. A high degree of exposure to alcohol in the early life of people who marry an alcoholic mate is fairly common.

Discussion of the sequencing of events surrounding alcohol use prior to and during the marriage is another crucial area. What was the courtship period like? When did the drinking become a problem? Did it predate the marriage or occur some time after the couple was wed? Has the drinker ever stopped drinking for a period of time? If so, what happened within the family at that time? If alcohol problems predate the marriage, it can be assumed that the couple has rarely talked, worked, made love, relaxed, or cared for their children without the ever-present specter of intoxication. The entire marital history of such a couple may be unpleasant and distorted.

When alcoholism postdates the beginning of marriage, careful assessment of its onset is necessary. Did alcoholism develop insidiously or was its onset more sudden and in response to some traumatic event?

All these questions and many more may need in-depth exploration, a task that goes beyond the initial appraisal by the nurse in a general health care setting. They are mentioned here to sensitize the nurse to the kinds of appraisal questions that need to be raised with the person who is close to one with alcoholism. The ultimate goal of the initial appraisal is to determine if indeed a problem exists and, if so, its nature and extent. Referral resources can then be suggested to the person who needs them. If the nurse possesses counseling skills, she may wish to engage the family member in this process.

Referral sources

The spouse, experiencing distress in her personal and family life as a result of living with an alcoholic mate, needs to know that she often needs treatment in her own right. Some spouses may find it difficult to accept this notion, having developed a pattern of allowing other family members' needs, especially those of the alcoholic person, to take priority over their own. Much energy often has been consumed in attempting to cope with the alcoholism and its disruptive effect on others, and spouses tend to place themselves in a secondary position.[14] Others may reject help, fearing that to do so would imply they are at fault or causing the problem. Discussing such beliefs, if they are present, will need to precede suggestions of where to go for help.

Al-Anon

There are several community support organizations available in most cities for spouses of alcoholic persons including Al-Anon, a self-help fellowship based on the principles of Alcoholics Anonymous. Al-Anon is tailored by and for the specific problems of spouses, relatives, and close friends of alcoholic persons. It was conceived in the late 1940s and has since grown rapidly so that now most communities have one or more Al-Anon chapters that meet on a regular basis.

Al-Anon meetings are warm, nonthreatening, and supportive. Friendships develop there that carry over into daily life. Regular telephone interaction occurs frequently between members at any hour of the day or night, whenever a member feels the need for immediate help or support.

The dynamics of the Al-Anon process works through a combination of educational and operational principles that the member must accept to change their behavior.[1] They include the didactic lesson that *alcoholism is a disease of the mind and the body and not a moral fault or perverse whim of the drinker*. Acceptance of the disease concept helps remove guilt, shame, and anger from the member.

In addition to the didactic lesson three operational principles, involving changes in attitudes and behavior, help members make Al-Anon work for them.[1] The first principle is *loving detachment from the alcoholic person*. This involves learning that it is not possible to control the actions of any person other than oneself. If members change their behavior, conditions may improve for them. The object of changing their behavior is to make life more enjoyable for themselves. The purpose is not to change the alcoholic person's behavior.

The second principle is *reestablishment of self-esteem and independence*. A chief goal of Al-Anon is to work on self-improvement. This is a luxury that most spouses have not taken advantage of for many years, since they have intensely focused on caring for the alcoholic mate.

The third principle *is reliance on a higher power*, which means achieving strength to make behavioral changes through spiritual means. For most members the higher power is God or Jesus, whereas for others it is the collective social support of the Al-Anon group or some other power of the member's own choosing.

The Al-Anon program provides a supportive peer group in which all members share a common problem. Through mutual aid members learn to change behavior and become involved in a recovery process tailored to meet their individual needs as persons close to an alcoholic person.

Nurses need to experience Al-Anon meetings firsthand by attending such a meeting in the community that is open to the general public. They need to become acquainted with when and where groups meet and to get to know several members and their telephone numbers for referral purposes. The value of using Al-Anon as a resource needs to be well understood by nurses and all professional workers who come in contact with family members of an alcoholic person.

Parents Anonymous

Some spouses of alcoholic mates, unable to find a suitable or safe outlet for their frustrations, vent them on their children. Whether frustrations are released through physical or verbal means, such a parent needs help in learning alternative ways of handling feelings. Parents Anonymous is another self-help group patterned after Alcoholics Anonymous that provides child-abusing parents with an opportunity to discuss common problems. Unlike Al-Anon and Alcoholics Anonymous, Parents Anonymous have professional sponsors. These sponsors, knowledgeable about child abuse, refer parents in need of treatment to additional sources of help.

Alcohol treatment centers

Most communities have outpatient community alcohol centers, sometimes called councils on alcoholism, which provide alcohol education through literature, speaker's bureaus, and short-term classes for special groups with alcohol-related problems. These centers are staffed to provide assessment, motivational counseling, and referral for both alcoholic persons and family members. They are an excellent first place to refer the spouse who wants to learn about the overall effects of alcohol and the variety of alcoholism treatment sources available in the community, and who may desire the opportunity to talk more about personal problems and where to go for further intervention.

In some instances the spouse might be referred for individual or group counseling along fairly traditional psychotherapy models in a community mental health center. The spouse also might receive counseling from an alcoholism specialist in private practice or one employed by an outpatient alcoholism center who will provide help in learning to cope with a mate's alcoholism.

A family approach to the treatment of alcoholism is becoming more widely practiced. This is coming about as treatment personnel become convinced of the need to help family members as well as the alcoholic person and become prepared to do so in a skillful manner. Thus in some communities the spouse and children might become involved in outpatient family therapy even before the alcoholic person is motivated to join them.

More and more inpatient alcohol centers are incorporating a systems approach and are treating the entire family rather than just dealing with the individual pathology of the drinker. When the whole family becomes involved, the emphasis is on improving family interaction and function as well as alleviating the alcoholism. Family therapy often needs to continue after sobriety has been achieved because of the occurrence of changing and continuing problems into this phase.

Spouses need to know that help is available to them, either through self-help organizations or through professional interventions found in formalized counseling agencies or through a combination of the two. They do not need to wait until the alcoholic person decides to receive help for a drinking problem. Much distress can be alleviated for spouses by their seeking and receiving help in their own right.

APPRAISAL OF CHILDREN

Until recently the needs of children of alcoholic parents have received relatively little attention as a subject of concern and systematic study by society. There exists a parallel lack of services designed to meet the special needs of these children. In spite of limited substantive findings based on well-designed research, there is a growing body of knowledge concerning the particular effect of parental alcoholism on children.[25] The nurse who is appraising the child will need to know these effects, be able to identify clues, promote a dialogue with the child, and make appropriate referrals. In these appraisal efforts the nurse needs to keep in mind that the drinking patterns of alcoholic persons vary enormously and therefore the degree and type of stress to which children are exposed within their families will vary also.

Effects of alcoholism on children

Emotional neglect by one or both parents is the most frequent problem experienced by children from alcoholic homes.[5, 10] These children have been called the "forgotten children" because their needs have been ignored so often.

Emotional neglect means that the child cannot communicate with his parent(s), he gets no emotional support from them, he does not get the feeling that they care about him as a person; the parents ignore the child's basic emotional needs, they do not make an effort to understand him, they spend little or no time with him, they give him no affection or warmth, they build a wall around themselves blocking any meaningful interaction.[5, p. 19]

Although physical neglect is identified less often as a problem, emotional neglect results from preoccupation by both parents with the alcoholism. The alcoholic parent's time and energy is largely consumed by drinking. When the father has alcoholism, he may do most of his drinking outside the home, being absent for long time periods. At home he may be drunk or hung over, isolated from the family, and incapacitated in the parental role. The alcoholic mother is more likely to drink at home. To hide her drinking, she too may isolate herself and allow the children undue amounts of freedom so as not to be disturbed.

Children living in alcoholic homes have difficulty understanding why their needs are seemingly of so little importance to their parents. The fact that the neglect is not willful does not lessen the devastation these children feel. It may take them a long time to realize that the reason for the neglect is related to something called alcoholism rather than to the fact that there is something deficient or bad about themselves.

In addition to emotional neglect, parents with alcohol-related problems are usually unable to provide a family atmosphere free of conflict. *Family conflict* involves violence, aggression, fighting, and arguments. The children experience, both as observers or direct participants, the parents' inept attempts to deal constructively with disagreements. They may overhear heated parental arguments and observe their parents hating and hurting one another. When the children witness physical abuse between their parents, they are likely to feel terrified. School phobia may relate to the child's wish to stay home and protect the parents from harming one another. Sometimes an older child in the family will imitate the parents by releasing pent-up feelings violently on a younger sibling, further complicating the home situation.

Families with alcoholism of one or both parents are at *high risk for abusive treatment of children*.[31] Physical abuse by parents results in injuries to children that include bruises, cuts, concussions, and broken bones. One of the key aspects of the hardship experienced by children in alcoholic homes may be violence. In situations where there is violence, children experience increased symptomatology—so much so that one might wonder if it is violence rather than alcoholism per se which is the important stress producing effects on the children.[32]

A severe form of abuse involves *sexual abuse* of the child by the parent. This problem is often unrevealed because the child is ashamed and fearful and does not tell anyone what has happened. Therefore accurate incidence rates are unavailable. Examples of sexual abuse that have been cited include a widowed alcoholic mother seductively caressing and rubbing against her adolescent daughter, the rape of an adolescent daughter by her alcoholic father, and a prepubescent son being periodically sodomized by an alcoholic father.[5]

Disturbances in role fulfillment are another consequence when a family member has alcoholism. It soon becomes evident that the alcoholic person cannot be relied on to perform expected roles consistently. To compensate, nonalcoholic members shift their role performance in an effort to keep the family functioning. The spouse often takes on additional responsibilities abdicated by the alcoholic partner. If the spouse fails to absorb these responsibilities, the burden may fall to the children who will then be expected to play roles and meet parental needs uncommon to other families.[19]

In some homes the nonalcoholic wife may encourage an older son to take over responsibilities renounced by the father, placing the son in an uncomfortable competitive role with his father. A different role shift may occur when the father has alcoholism and there is a teenage daughter. As problems increase in her relationship with her husband, the mother may gradually relinquish her role as wife, inadvertently setting her daughter up to assume that role. When the father is sober and trying to make restitution, he may present his daughter with gifts or give her special attention. This can be highly confusing to the daughter in the throes of adolescence who is involved in working out feelings about her own sexuality and relationships with the opposite sex. Sometimes the daughter concludes that her father prefers her to the mother. She may fantasize that if her mother were more loving, her father would not drink. Such a girl may grow up and marry an alcoholic man, believing she is capable of curing his ills with love, only to fail in these efforts.

Neither parent can provide their children with good *role models* of healthy adult behavior. The alcoholic parent behaves inconsistently and unpredictably. Depending on the state of intoxication, the alcoholic person's behavior may vary from dull to gregarious or from gentle to abusive. The nonalcoholic parent, in turn, often fails to demonstrate healthy patterns of response to stress. Children often criticize the nonalcoholic parent's coping behavior, noticing, for example, that nagging accomplishes little. Some children believe that the sober parent should use better judgment in the way he or she behaves, since the alcoholic parent seems less responsible.

Both parents are likely to present confusing models of behavior in other areas as well. The alcoholic father often lies about his drinking, minimizing the amount or that he has been drinking at all. The nonalcoholic mother may call the father's place of employment to alibi his absence from work. She fabricates that he has the flu or that there has been a death in the family, when the children know he is in a nearby bedroom drunk or hung over. Both parents, however, punish the children for lying.

Children growing up in a home with an alcoholic parent will no doubt find it *difficult to emulate either parent*. The nonalcoholic parent may appear strong and dependable but joyless. The alcoholic parent appears needy and weak but more carefree. Such circumstances provide a growing child with few opportunities for healthy role identification within the family unit.

Another important area in child and adolescent development that suffers when a parent has alcoholism concerns *friendship formation*.[32] Children from alcoholic homes often have trouble making friends for various reasons. The difficulty may be related to the alcoholic parent's not allowing other children in the home or ordering them out of the house when they do visit. More often it involves the child's feeling of reciprocity in friendship. Because of shame and embarrassment, children with alcoholic parents do not want to return invitations to others who have invited them to their homes. They do not want their friends to see the alcoholic parent drunk or to witness family arguments and discord. Thus they cease initiating activities with friends or potential friends that require parental support and involvement, and with time the child is no longer invited to visit outside the home. Friendships therefore are less likely to flourish, and the child experiences social isolation from peers.

Finally, children of alcoholic parents are especially *vulnerable to developing alcoholism* later in their own lives. It has been predicted that as many as 58% of future alcoholic populations will be derived from children of alcoholic parents.[6] Through exposure to adults who rely heavily on alcohol for anxiety reduction and to mass media that encourage alcohol use as part of the "good life," many children of alcoholic parents gain powerful impressions about the importance of future use of alcohol in their own lives. Such children may be so reinforced and patterned toward excessive alcohol use that the outcome is certain.[8]

Children's response

Children's feelings about living with an alcoholic parent derive from the particular situations they experience and their perception of them. In turn, their feelings influence how they cope with their problems.

Although children experience and express a full range of emotions toward an alcoholic parent, the most common feelings are *resentment* and *embarrassment*.[5] They resent the neglect and conflict, the absence of the alcoholic person, and being forced to carry heavy adult responsibilities. Children are embarrassed by the parent's dependency, social inadequacies, and nonfulfillment of parental responsibility. Other feelings children express include love, respect, fear, anger and hate, guilt, and loneliness. Most of the feelings are negative, and there is a great deal of ambivalence toward the alcoholic parent among these children.

As stated previously, parental alcoholism is not equally disruptive in all families, and some children have a compensatory relationship with a grandparent, teacher, or neighbor that assists them to cope with the alcoholism of a parent. Many children find ways of developing constructive, appropriate defenses, whereas others need not take extreme measures to defend themselves because the situation is not seriously disruptive.

Four predominant coping or defense patterns have been described for children from homes with alcoholism. The patterns are categorized as flight, fight, perfect child, and super-coper syndrome.[5]

The most common pattern is *flight*, in which the child escapes. The escape varies and can be physical, mental, or emotional. The young child may hide from the alcoholic parent under a bed, whereas older children spend long hours away from home. Other children may gradually deaden their emotions by becoming cold and hard.

Fight involves rebellion, verbal and physical aggression, acting out, and socially unacceptable behavior. Children usually learn that the price for fight is too high, since it often increases the aggressiveness of the parent toward the child. It may be used a few times and then abandoned.

The *perfect child* tries to be good all the time by not doing anything. He does not give anyone any trouble by being obedient and passive. He avoids incurring anyone's wrath so that he will not be hurt.

The *super-coper* is actively attempting to do everything right. He tries to handle every problem for the family, comforting his mother about her husband's drinking or working to pay family bills. He is sometimes known as the family saviour.

A few children are unable to find a way to cope and so they remain *victimized*. They may suffer learning disorders, psychosis, or brain damage and live out their lives in institutions or foster homes.

Clues to presence of parental alcoholism

A review of the findings of studies done on children from alcoholic homes indicates that these children are likely to display behavior or conduct problems. *Temper tantrums, fighting with peers, trouble in school* including *unacceptable conduct and truancy*, and *involvement with police and courts* are among the findings from several of these studies.[9, 17]

Children with an alcoholic parent are often *reared* in *unstable or broken homes* and have *negative attitudes toward authority*.[30] Their *self-esteem* may be *low* and their *trust* and *confidence* in others *poorly developed*. They may have *difficulty establishing friendships* with peers and be *socially isolated*. *Burdened by an inordinate amount of responsibility at home, they lack time and energy for socializing with others*. Because of their *high-risk status* for *physical abuse*, these children may show signs such as excessive bruises or broken bones with vague explanation as to the cause.

The problems encountered by children from families with alcoholism are probably not substantially different from those of children from any unhappy home. However, the *progression of symptoms may be more rapid and pronounced and behavior patterns more predictable*, often reflecting the drinking pattern of the alcoholic parent. For example, if the parent is a weekend drinker, the child may be depressed on Monday, improve during the week, and display extreme anxiety by the end of the week. If the parent is a periodic drinker, the child is likely to display symptoms at those times when the parent is drinking.[13]

When the nurse suspects that a child may be living in a home with alcoholism, it is important to initiate questions that will further clarify the situation. In doing so, the nurse hopes to obtain adequate appraisal data to develop plans for intervention that are responsive to the child's needs.

Promoting a dialogue

Children from alcoholic homes may need particular assistance in describing and comprehending alcoholism and its impact on their lives. The nurse may be the one adult person to whom a troubled child can turn.

In an interview study involving 115 children, one or both of whose parents were alcoholic, it was found that once these children understood that an outsider was interested in them, they overcame their initial reluctance to share their concerns.[10] The children were eased into conversation by giving verbal recognition to their feelings by means of remarks such as, "I know it must be difficult to talk about something that upsets you so much." Being accessible and providing a nonjudgmental listening ear can be vital behavior by the nurse in promoting a dialogue. Most children will be able to share pertinent appraisal information if provided with a responsive atmosphere, and they will no doubt gain satisfaction and a sense of release from talking with the nurse about a subject that is usually taboo. In fact, in the interview study just mentioned, it was as though a "dam had burst" for a good many of the children once they began to talk.

Although each nurse will need to develop her own specific appraisal questions and *effective ways of phrasing them for individual children,* a few general questions that are usually appropriate and useful for children from alcoholic homes are suggested. These questions, presented in the following list, involve discovering the child's perceptions concerning what is happening at home, at school, and in regard to self.

Home

Are there any troubles in your home with alcohol?
In your opinion, whom in your family drinks too much?
How does your father/mother act when drunk? When sober?
How does your father/mother act when your mother/father is drunk?
What do you do when your father/mother is drunk?
How do you feel toward each of your parents?
Are you able to talk about your problems with your parents?
Do you have brothers, sisters, or close relatives nearby whom you like and whom you
　　can talk with?
What do you do with your family that is fun?
What responsibilities do you have at home?
Do you invite friends to your home?

School

How do you get along with your teachers?
How do you get along with your classmates?
What kind of grades do you get in school?
Are you able to concentrate on your schoolwork?
Are there any adults at school you could talk over your problems with, like a coun-
　　selor, nurse, or teacher?
Do you participate in any extra activities, like sports, drama, or music?

Self

How do you feel about yourself?
Do you have any problems letting others know what you are really like?
How do you go about making new friends?
Do you have any trouble keeping friends?
How do you get attention from others?
Does anything worry you?
Are you afraid of anything?

In general, the nurse needs to assess the nature and the extent of the effect of parental alcoholism on the child and how the child is dealing with it. Ways of strengthening the child's coping ability may need to be found as well as ways of building additional support systems. When there is emotional or physical neglect or abuse, community resources must be identified to provide appropriate help for the child.

Support systems and community resources

Resources for children of alcoholic parents need to assist the children to survive in their environments, provide them with compensatory love and care, strengthen their coping abilities, and further their individual growth and development. The resources may be individuals or community agencies and organizations.

Individuals

There may be individuals within the nuclear or extended family who can intervene by counterbalancing some of the deficiencies found in the child's home. The nuclear or extended family, however, can only be a resource if its members are truly concerned and available to the child. Most persons are capable of increasing their support when they are mobilized to do so. Some may need to receive outside guidance and understanding themselves regarding alcoholism to be consistently responsive to the needs of a child.

Nurses, physicians, counselors, teachers, and members of the clergy are all persons within the community who can potentially be of help to children from alcoholic homes. To be effective, they may need to develop a heightened awareness and understanding of the experiences and needs of these children. At a minimum, to be a potential resource, professional people need to be able to recognize problems of alcohol abuse in a family, provide short-term counseling, and connect the child with other needed resources.

Alateen

Alateen, an affiliate of Alcoholics Anonymous, is the principal community resource available nationwide to children, primarily teenagers, who have a parent, relative, or friend who has alcoholism. Alatot for younger children has developed in a few isolated urban areas. In Alateen the children learn that alcoholism is a family disease, with persons being responsible for their own recovery. Children concentrate in Alateen on their personal growth to lessen the harmful effects of alcoholism on their lives.[2]

Alateen groups, found in most large cities, have adult sponsors, usually from Al-Anon or sometimes from Alcoholics Anonymous. The sponsors are responsible for developing and maintaining the Alateen groups. They are present at meetings and sometimes make themselves available to the children on a one-to-one basis.

It is the peer group who provides a sensitive environment where the child can talk about problems associated with parental alcoholism. As in Al-Anon and Alcoholics Anonymous, children in Alateen learn to rely on a higher power to help them understand alcoholism and to develop a greater sense of personal strength. Alateen is unable to provide for all the needs of the child. For those who can accept its tenets and approach, Alateen offers help primarily through peer support. There are no dues or fees for services, making it financially feasible for any child.

Children's protective services

Children from alcoholic homes who experience abuse, neglect, or exploitation will need assistance from Children's Protective Services. Case workers are available within these services to investigate such situations and to assist the child and the family with rehabilitation. Temporary and permanent foster homes and adoption services are also available. Parents may directly seek assistance, or outside reports of neglect or abuse may activate agency intervention. Although programs vary, all states have laws making it mandatory for any person knowing about incidents of child abuse, neglect, or exploitation to report them.

Legally, children may not seek or receive services or treatment without parental consent, with the exception of protective services for abuse and neglect. A legal trend with respect to children and treatment is the tendency to allow new levels of independence for children.[29] There is a general need for opening treatment options for children independently of considerations of parental consent. This may be especially necessary for children from alcoholic homes whose parents are sometimes unwilling or unable to see the need for seeking outside help for their children.

Alcoholism treatment programs

Alcoholism treatment programs provide limited services for children for several reasons.[5] First, most of these programs focus primarily on the alcoholic person, and when nonalcoholic family members are included, it is most often only the spouse. Second, family members mainly make contact with alcoholism programs when the alcoholic person decides to receive treatment. Since the percentage of alcoholic persons in treatment is small, the possibility of a child's being in treatment is proportionately meager. Third, some of these programs are located at a distance from the family, creating a financial burden that is difficult, if not impossible, for the family members to deal with. Fourth, many alcoholism counselors lack education and experience in responding to the needs of children and may believe that the recovery of the alcoholic parent is all that the child needs.

Although few options other than Alateen are available in most communities to meet the special needs of this group of children, isolated programs have been developed and implemented. One such program involved an eight-session workshop for children whose fathers were alcoholic and for their nonalcoholic mothers.[27] The overall goal of the workshop was to promote adaptive communication between participants. This education/prevention effort made use of techniques such as role playing with hand puppets, artwork consisting of construction of a collage of the drinking member of the family, and composing poetry or prose using words such as alcoholism, love, hate, lonely, mother, father, child. The effort produced some distinctly beneficial changes in the participants, especially for the mothers, but no dramatic results. A modified program is being planned to settle eventually on the most effective treatment program.

Clearly a great deal needs to be done for children from families with alcoholism. A major national effort needs to be launched to include all levels of intervention: prevention, early identification, and treatment. Many more agencies need to explore alternative approaches to identify the most efficacious interventions. Finally, nurses in diverse settings need to be inventive as they identify and, when needed, devise support systems and interventions within their own communities that are responsive to children from alcoholic homes.

REFERENCES

1. Ablon, J.: Al-Anon family groups, American Journal of Psychotherapy **28**:30, 1974.
2. Alateen, hope for children of alcoholics, New York, 1973, Al-Anon Family Group Headquarters, Inc.
3. Alger, I.: Audio-visual techniques in family therapy. In Bloch, D. A., editor: Techniques of family psychotherapy, New York, 1973, Grune & Stratton, Inc.
4. Bloch, D. A., and LaPerriere, K.: Techniques of family therapy: a conceptual frame. In Bloch, D. A., editor: Techniques of family psychotherapy, New York, 1973, Grune & Stratton, Inc.
5. Booz-Allen, and Hamilton, Inc.: An assessment of the needs of and resources for children of alcoholic parents, PB-241 119, Rockville, Md., 1974, National Institute of Alcohol Abuse and Alcoholism.
6. Bosma, W. G. A.: Alcoholism and teenagers, Maryland State Medical Journal **24**:62, 1975.
7. Bowen, M.: Alcoholism as viewed through family systems theory and family psychotherapy. In Seixas, F. A., et al., editors: The person with alcoholism, Annals of the New York Academy of Sciences **233**:115, 1974.
8. Burk, E. D.: Some contemporary issues in child development and the children of alcoholic parents, Annals of the New York Academy of Sciences **197**:189, 1972.
9. Chafetz, M. E., Blane, H. T., and Hill, M. J.: Children of alcoholics: observations in the child-guidance clinic, Quarterly Journal of Studies on Alcohol **32**:687, 1971.
10. Cork, R. M.: The forgotten children, Toronto, 1969, Addiction Research Foundation of Ontario.
11. Crosby, M. H.: Control systems and children with lymphoblastic leukemia, Nursing Clinics of North America **6**:407, 1971.
12. Estes, N. J.: Counseling the wife of an alcoholic spouse, American Journal of Nursing **74**:1251, 1974.
13. Estes, N. J., and Hanson, K. J.: Alcoholism in the family: prespectives for the nurse practitioner, Nurse Practitioner **1**:125, 1976.

14. Estes, N. J., and Hanson, K. J.: Sobriety: problems, challenges, and solutions, American Journal of Psychotherapy **30:**256, 1976.
15. Finlay, D. G.: Anxiety and the alcoholic, Social Work **17:**29, 1972.
16. Gorad, S. L., McCourt, W. F., and Cobb, J. C.: A communications approach to alcoholism, Quarterly Journal of Studies on Alcohol **32:**651, 1971.
17. Haberman, P. W.: Childhood symptoms in children of alcoholics and comparison group parents, Journal of Marriage and the Family **28:**152, 1966.
18. Hazzard, M. E.: An overview of systems theory, Nursing Clinics of North America **6:**385, 1971.
19. Hecht, M.: Children of alcoholics are children at risk, American Journal of Nursing **73:**1764, 1973.
20. Howard, D., and Howard, N.: The family 20-question questionnaire, 1976, Box 1362, Columbia, Mo. 65201.
21. Jackson, J. K.: The adjustment of the family to the crisis of alcoholism, Quarterly Journal of Studies on Alcohol **15:**562, 1954.
22. Jackson, J. K.: The adjustment of the family to alcoholism, Marriage and the Family **18:**361, 1956.
23. Jackson, J. K.: Family structure and alcoholism, Mental Hygiene **43:**403, 1959.
24. Jackson, J. K.: Alcoholism and the family. In Pittman, D. J., and Snyder, C. R., editors: Society, culture and drinking patterns, New York, 1962, John Wiley & Sons, Inc.
25. Jacob, T., et al.: The alcoholic's spouse, children and family interactions, Journal of Studies on Alcohol **39:**1231, 1978.
26. James, J. E., and Goldman, M.: Behavior trends of wives of alcoholics, Quarterly Journal of Studies on Alcohol **32:**373, 1971.
27. Kern, J. C., et al.: A treatment approach for children of alcoholics, Journal of Drug Education **7:**207, 1977-78.
28. Lederer, W. J., and Jackson, D. D.: The mirages of marriage, New York, 1968, W. W. Norton & Co., Inc., Publishers.
29. McCabe, J.: Children in need: consent issues in treatment, Alcohol Health and Research World **2:**2, 1977.
30. Mik, G.: Sons of alcoholic fathers, British Journal of Addiction **65:**305, 1970.
31. Olson, R. J.: Index of suspicion: screening for child abusers, American Journal of Nursing **76:**108, 1976.
32. Orford, J.: Impact of alcoholism on family and home. In Edwards, G., and Grant, M., editors: Alcoholism: new knowledge and new responses, London, 1977, Croom Helm Ltd.
33. Orford, J., et al.: The role of excessive drinking in alcoholism complicated marriages: a study of stability and change over a one-year period, International Journal of the Addictions **12:**471, 1977.
34. Orford, J., and Guthrie, S.: Coping behavior used by wives of alcoholics: a preliminary investigation. (Abstract.) In Proceedings of the 28th International Congress on Alcohol and Alcoholism, Washington, D.C., 1968, Program Publications Committee, International Congress on Alcohol and Alcoholism.
35. Paolina, T. J., and McCrady, B. S.: The alcoholic marriage: alternative perspectives, New York, 1977, Grune & Stratton, Inc.
36. Satir, V.: People making, Palo Alto, Calif., 1972, Science & Behavior Books, Inc.
37. 22 questions that can help decide if someone close has a drinking problem: Reflect, June, 1977, Dallas, Dallas Council on Alcoholism.
38. Ward, R. F., and Faillace, L. A.: The alcoholic and his helpers: a systems view, Quarterly Journal of Studies on Alcohol **31:**684, 1970.

Index